FLUID AND BLOOD THERAPY IN ANESTHESIA

FLUID AND BLOOD THERAPY IN ANESTHESIA

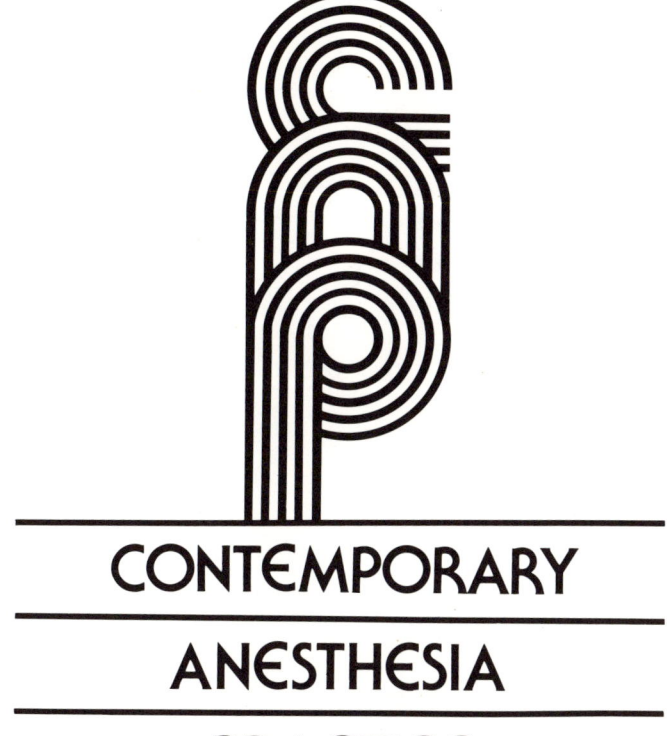

CONTEMPORARY

ANESTHESIA

PRACTICE

BURNELL R. BROWN, JR., EDITOR
CASEY D. BLITT & A. H. GIESECKE, ASSOCIATE EDITORS

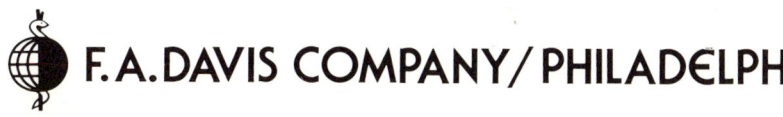

F. A. DAVIS COMPANY/PHILADELPHIA

Copyright © 1983 by F. A. Davis Company

All rights reserved. This book is protected by copyright. No part of it may be reproduced, stored in a retrieval system, or transmitted in any form or by any means, electronic, mechanical, photocopying, recording, or otherwise, without written permission from the publisher.

Printed in the United States of America

Library of Congress Cataloging in Publication Data
Main entry under title:

Fluid and blood therapy in anesthesia.

  (Contemporary anesthesia practice ; v. 6)
  Includes bibliographical references and index.
  1. Therapeutics, Surgical. 2. Fluid therapy. 3. Blood—Transfusion. 4. Anesthesia—Complications and sequelae. I. Brown, Burnell R. II. Series.
  [DNLM: 1. Anesthesia. 2. Fluid therapy. 3. Water-electrolyte balance. 4. Blood transfusion. 5. Intraoperative care.
W1 C07969ME v.6 / WO 181 F646]
RD52.F59F59   1983   617'.96   82-10075
ISBN 0-8036-1273-7

PREFACE

This volume of *Contemporary Anesthesia Practice* is devoted to a discussion of several issues concerning blood and fluid use. It is not proposed to offer a comprehensive review of all facets of the subject within these covers. Rather, a number of appropriate topics have been condensed for presentation to the reader.

Intraoperative fluid therapy frequently generates more heat than light on the firing line of the operating room. The era of strong resistance to the use of salt-containing solutions seems to have passed, but misconceptions nonetheless remain. As an example, I have more than once heard the admonition: "Do not give Ringer's lactate, as this patient is shocky and already has a lactic acid acidosis." What an inexcusable offense against the science of chemistry! Lactate ion is not lactic acid. Lactate ion by itself is a base, pure and simple, capable of formidable amounts of hydrogen ion buffering. In truth, when hapatic perfusion becomes adequate, lactate, a three-carbon compound, can eventually be metabolized into three molecules of bicarbonate. The concern is not lactic acid buildup and metabolic acidosis; it is metabolic alkalosis enhancement. The role of albumin and indications for its use form another area of great misunderstanding.

Component blood therapy is much maligned by surgeon and anesthesiologist alike. Yet there are manifold virtues to this type of replacement, and few vices if proper administration and rationale are employed. It is shocking that dilution of packed red cells with Ringer's lactate continues to occur. Calcium in the balanced salt solution is sufficient to deactivate every bit of the citrate anticoagulant so that rouleaux formation and sludging occur. This and other points of component therapy are discussed in the text that follows.

I wish to express my thanks to the authors of the various chapters for tasks well done. As always, this brief volume is dedicated to the safety of our patients.

Burnell R. Brown, Jr.

CONTRIBUTORS

R. Dennis Bastron, M.D.
Associate Professor of Anesthesiology
University of Arizona College of Medicine
Tucson, Arizona

Charles A. Baxter, M.D.
Frank H. Kidd, Jr. Professor of Surgery
University of Texas
Health Science Center at Dallas
Dallas, Texas

Frederic A. Berry, M.D.
Professor of Anesthesiology and Pediatrics
University of Virginia Medical Center
Charlottesville, Virginia

Burnell R. Brown, Jr., M.D., Ph.D.
Professor and Chairman
Department of Anesthesiology
University of Arizona College of Medicine
Tucson, Arizona

Jerry M. Calkins, M.D.
Assistant Professor of Anesthesiology
University of Arizona College of Medicine
Tucson, Arizona

C. James Carrico, M.D.
Professor and Chief
Department of Surgery
Harborview Hospital
Seattle, Washington

Robert E. Drake, Ph.D.
Associate Professor of Anesthesiology
University of Texas
Health Science Center
Houston, Texas

Joseph C. Gabel, M.D.
Professor and Chairman
Department of Anesthesiology
University of Texas
Health Science Center
Houston, Texas

Douglas W. Huestis, M.D.
Professor of Pathology
Chief, Immunohematology
University of Arizona College of Medicine
Tucson, Arizona

Robert R. Kirby, M.D.
Chariman, Department of Anesthesiology
Wilford Hall USAF Medical Center
Lackland AFB, Texas

M. T. Jenkins, M.D.
McDermott Professor
Department of Anesthesiology
University of Texas
Southwestern Medical School at Dallas
Dallas, Texas

Ronald V. Maier, M.D.
Assistant Professor of Surgery
Harborview Hospital
Seattle, Washington

George H. Rodman, Jr., M.D.
Director of Trauma Services
Good Samaritan Medical Center
Phoenix, Arizona

Reynolds J. Saunders, M.D.
Instructor of Anesthesiology
University of Arizona College of Medicine
Tucson, Arizona

Karen Steinbronn, M.D.
Assistant Professor of Pathology
University of Arizona College of Medicine
Chief, Hematopathology
Veterans Administration Medical Center
Tucson, Arizona

CONTENTS

1. HISTORY OF ACUTE SEQUESTERED EDEMA IN SURGERY AND TRAUMA   1
   M. T. Jenkins, M.D.

2. SODIUM BALANCE   33
   R. Dennis Bastron, M.D.

3. BALANCED SALT SOLUTIONS IN MASSIVE TRAUMA   57
   C. James Carrico, M.D., and Ronald V. Maier, M.D.

4. INTRAOPERATIVE FLUID THERAPY IN PEDIATRICS   85
   Frederic A. Berry, M.D.

5. ROLE OF COLLOID OSMOTIC PRESSURE IN SHOCK AND RESUSCITATION   5
   Robert E. Drake, Ph.D., and Joseph C. Gable, M.D.

6. POST-TRAUMATIC RESPIRATORY FAILURE: ROLE OF FLUID THERAPY   119
   George H. Rodman, Jr., M.D, and Robert R. Kirby, M.D.

7. BALANCED SALT SOLUTIONS AS RENAL PROPHYLAXIS   137
   Charles A. Baxter, M.D.

8. RATIONALE FOR BLOOD COMPONENT THERAPY   151
   Karen Sreinbronn, M.D, and Douglas W. Huestis, M.D.

9. PRACTICAL CONSIDERATIONS IN TRANSFUSION TECHNIQUES DURING ANESTHESIA   169
   Reynolds J. Saunders, M.D., and Jerry M. Calkins, M.D., Ph.D.

INDEX   183

HISTORY OF SEQUESTERED EDEMA ASSOCIATED WITH SURGICAL OPERATIONS AND TRAUMA

M. T. Jenkins, M.D.

I recall the maxim current during my medical student days: "Do not administer even one milliequivalent of sodium during surgery and for 48 hours postoperatively." Obviously there have been radical changes in the philosophy of fluid and electrolyte therapy since the era of obligate sodium retention. Dr. Jenkins is certainly one of the best qualified physicians to recount the tale of the no-salt-to-salt pendulum swing. He was on the "ground floor" in Dr. Carl Moyer's Surgery Department, where the concept of considering the interstitial extracellular fluid space of surgical patients first developed. He was a contemporary and coworker with Moyer, Wilson, Shires, Seldon, and others who contributed vital knowledge to our understanding of the dynamics of fluid shifts in the surgical and trauma patient.

In this historical overview, Dr. Jenkins goes back further, however. His discrediting of the Woods and Pravaz title to syringe and needle invention is both interesting and iconoclastic. He describes Rudolph Matas' use of saline solutions in the late nineteenth century. Dr. Matas contributed in many areas of anesthesia-related care, and was the first physician in the U.S. to administer spinal anesthesia. Rumor has it that his use of saline infusions in his surgical patients was based on his penchant for eating watermelons liberally laced with salt following a morning of surgery in the hot, humid environment of old Charity Hospital's unairconditioned operating rooms in New Orleans!

Dr. Jenkins' remarkable contribution is especially noteworthy because of his incisively annotated references. This article is a delight to read.

Burnell R. Brown, Jr.

PROLOGUE

The importance of the translocation of extracellular fluid from the dynamics of the circulation has developed over the past three decades, while knowledge of the circulation of blood and the consequent infusion of intravenous fluids dates back three and one-half centuries.

In this review of intravenous fluid administration three events in the remote past are labeled epochal: Harvey's description of the circulation of the blood (1628),[1,2] Lister's proposal of the germ theory (1875),[11] and Bernard's physiologic treatise on the milieu internus (1879).[12] A fourth epoch began in the recent past with Shires' publication in 1959 of the concisely detailed work, *Changing Concept of Salt Water and Surgery*.[73] In this and in subsequent publications, Shires and his associates have established that the extracellular fluid (ECF) has a large functional component and is a mobile and measurable pool. In this documented concept the ECF responds rapidly to a variety of stimuli, including blood loss without significant trauma, both hemorrhage and trauma, trauma without blood loss, and many illnesses.[77]

Knowledge of the ECF is not recent, of course. Bernard appreciated it as the immediate environment of the organism.[12] Gamble, in a delightful lecture on the extracellular fluid and its vicissitudes, presented an excellent description of the ECF as an anatomic force, largely stationary, lending stability to physico-chemical conditions within the organism.[49]

As new information has developed and as practices of perioperative fluid management have changed, beliefs in the inevitable results of surgical trauma have been revised. No longer is it thought that anesthesia and operation invariably cause renal intolerance to salt or renal inability to excrete administered salt. Nor is hyponatremia or oliguria expected as a result only of anesthesia and surgical trauma. Based on current knowledge of sequestered edema, when hyponatremia and oliguria occurred in the past, the etiology was more likely to be failure to administer balanced salt solutions sufficient to replace that lost from the dynamics of the circulation. ECF can be lost through translocation into edema sites, and perhaps also into muscle cells, as has been explored by Shires and associates.

Our appreciation of fluid shifts today will be enhanced by a review of the history of beliefs and practices in fluid administration.

Inasmuch as no critical historical review of intravenous infusions is available, I will offer one here, with references and discussion relating to the evolution in attitudes and practices. Many of the historical references contain a precis, frequently with a direct quotation and occasionally with a critical comment.

REMOTE HISTORY (1628–1899)

Intravenous injection of drugs and fluids became a rational procedure after 1628, the year William Harvey published his findings on the circulation of the blood. Interestingly, the treatise in Latin was printed and published at Frankfurt-on-Main, then considered a center of learning more fitting than London to receive such an important review of his anatomic exercises. It was addressed to "Charles, King of Great Britain, France, and Ireland," and was titled *Exercitatio Anatomica de Motu Cordis et Sanguinis in Animalibus.*[1,2]

In translation, the opening sentence of the dedication to the king sets the central theme of his experiments: "The heart of creatures is the foundation of life, the Prince of all, the Sun of their microcosm, on which all vegetation does depend, from whence all vigor and strength does flow."

Harvey is usually designated the discoverer of the circulation of the blood, suggesting that he stumbled suddenly and unexpectedly upon the truth when knowledge of bodily functions was still fettered by a blind belief in the teachings of great writers such as Aristotle and Galen. However, for 12 years, from about 1616, Harvey had been propounding his views in lectures and demonstrations at the Royal College of Physicians and probably had put them into practice in his wards at St. Bartholomew's Hospital.

Despite erroneous beliefs concerning functions of the heart and blood vessels prior to Harvey's epochal revelations, there is a recording of what is perhaps the earliest blood administration (a transfusion?) to Pope Innocent VIII in 1492. The recipient and the three boys used as donors all died. More than a century elapsed before transfusions were again alluded to, this time by De Colle of Padua in 1628, the year of Harvey's publication.[14]

The history of intravenous infusions is closely tied to the subject of injection of drugs. Probably the first experiments of this kind were performed in England, and not by a medical man. It was Christopher Wren, mathematician and later an architect (St. Paul's Cathedral) and an astronomer (Savilian Professor of Astronomy at Oxford), who at age 25 first tried the bold experiments of injecting drugs into the veins of animals. In the year 1656, using an apparatus consisting of a quill attached to a small bladder, he injected dogs with opium and with crocus mettallorum. The opium stupified the animals and the second drug produced violent vomiting.[3] The first intravenous injection of a drug in man probably was also by Wren, in 1657, using vinum emiticum.

A neglected contributor to the experiments on intravenous injections and infusions in the 17th Century is Johann Sigismund Elsholtz, state physician to the Great Elector of Berlin. In 1661 he wrote, "If a tankard of wine is poured into a river, the wine, together with the water flows into the sea. In just the same way whatever liquid is injected into a vein must necessarily reach the heart, together with the circulating blood."[4]

Elsholtz was intrigued with the new art of injecting solutions into veins so he wrote that it was not improper to label the procedure as "The New Clyster," combining the word clysis, the washing out of a cavity, with the Greek word, klyster, a syringe. His reference came to be the new clyster, or the art of the enema applied to arteries and veins by injecting through a syringe and needle.

Only a few years separated Harvey's publication on the circulation (1628) from Wren's intravenous injection of drugs (1657) and Elsholtz's Clysmatica Nova, the New Clyster (1667). Many decades then elapsed before the next significant studies, when practicing physicians played active roles in developing the physiology of body fluids. These developments were intimately related to the treatment of diseases, cholera (1831), diabetic coma (1874), and infantile diarrhea (1915–16).

In 1831, O'Shaughnessy analyzed the blood of patients with cholera and described changes showing that a large proportion of water was lost, neutral saline ingredients were lost, free alkali had disappeared, urine was suppressed, and urea was increased, although the globular structure of the blood remained unchanged. He proposed a new method of treating the epidemic cholera by the injection of large volumes of "highly-oxygenized salts" into the venous system.[5]

O'Shaughnessy recognized in his proposal of therapy that venesection, the standard of the age, might possibly help oxygenate arterial blood, but he rejected this modality along with oxygen plus atmospheric air, or oxygen with "the protoxide of azote, that singular aerial compound, to which the name of 'laughing gas' has been applied."
" . . . I propose . . . injection of powerful oxygenating salts directly into the veins . . . the tube which should be of gold or ivory, be introduced into the jugular vein . . . free from the entrance of air caused by the

suction force of the right side of the heart. . . ." Obviously O'Shaughnessy was aware of the several studies in France on air embolism published first in 1773 and continuing there as late as 1829.[23]

Lewins[6] and Latta[7] in separate letters in *Lancet* reported great success in treating cholera patients with salt solutions they had individually concocted from various formulae. Treatment was vigorous. As one example, Lewins described a patient he feared would die before he could begin injecting the salt solution. "Between seven at night and two o'clock next morning, there were thrown in 284 ounces, upwards of twenty-three pounds . . . a change for the better that appears almost miraculous has taken place."

As described by Moyer,[71] the use of salt solutions in medicine, except as purgatives, had to await the coming of analytic chemistry and the application of its methods to the study of the changes in blood that accompany disease. In 1831 O'Shaughnessy analyzed the blood of patients with cholera and based his treatment on his analysis. He mastered a lesson which has periodically been revived only to fade from use repeatedly in the history of fluid administration.

As knowledge of the epidemic of 1831 faded, the efficacy of saline therapy in cholera was forgotten in England. When cholera reappeared in London in epidemic form 20 years later, the lessons from O'Shaughnessy, Lewins, and Latta were not recalled, although they had been published in a prominent journal. Galenic treatment—bleeding, sweating, and purging—became the mode again with the predictable dire results.

Forty-three years after the chemical changes in cholera were described, Fagge in 1874 employed those earlier observations in the treatment of diabetic coma.[10]

At this point, it seems appropriate to mention the third disease which brought practicing physicians into active roles in developing the physiology of body fluids. In 1915 it was recognized that another deadly disease, infantile diarrhea, had many of the features of cholera. As noted by Moyer,[71] pediatricians have been pre-eminent in the field of fluid balance since the stimulating work by Holt, Courtney, and Fales in 1915,[19] and by Howland and Marriott in 1916[20] in fluid therapy with salt solutions to restore circulatory dynamics of infants ravaged by diarrhea.

It has been of historical interest to anesthesiologists in particular to place a date on the invention of the syringe and needle and their introduction into clinical practice. Various reports have set the dates in the mid-1800s when A. Wood of Scotland, F. Rynd of Ireland, C. G.

Pravaz of France, and Luer of France were involved in development and disputation of various instruments to inoculate drugs beneath the skin. As concluded by Howard-Jones, who noted that assertions about hypodermic medication varied from vague generalities to specific inaccuracies, there was no such invention as the syringe. It just happened.[65] (Note references above to Elsholtz, who recorded use of the syringe [and needle] in 1667.)

As the origin of hypodermic medication, including intravenous infusions, was pre-Listerian, none of the early practitioners had particular reasons for anticipating septic complications. When sepsis did occur it seems to have been ascribed to the patient's disease for which treatment was in progress. Charles Hunter, a house surgeon at St. George's, London, addressed the question of abscess or diffuse inflammation after the use of syringe and needle for hypodermic injections or infusions. "I have seen no ill effect of any kind from the puncture."[9]

A second epochal event in the history of intravenous infusions occurred in 1875 with the publication of Lister's germ theory, though it was not recognized as epochal at that time, when sepsis was thought to be part of the natural course of diseases being treated. Abscesses were explained as caused by using the same puncture site too often, or in the absence of multiple skin penetrations, to the roughness of the trocar or needle. No great argument is required today, however, to establish Lister as the father of antisepsis. The question of sterility of intravenous solutions developed many years after the germ theory became circulated and accepted.[11]

Only four years after Lister's disclosures, in 1879, a third epochal event occurred as Claude Bernard, a giant among 19th Century physiologists, wrote of "that bit of primeval sea within us."[12] He described it as the milieu internus or the internal environment, the true medium in which we live, so isolated from the world that atmospheric disturbances cannot alter it or penetrate beyond it. Nearly all studies of the complex biochemical system of the patient relate to the internal milieu described by Bernard and to the attainment of the state of balance known by the happy term, homeostasis. Since Bernard's publication the human body has been described as a delicately balanced system involving fluids, hormones, and electrolytes, recognizing that the individual cannot be freed of an aquatic heritage. Behind any consideration of fluid and electrolyte therapy for the patient lies the realization that the human body is made up of a collection of semipermeable sacs in which its semipermeable cells are bathed in fluid. Semipermeable membranes separate its capillaries, connective tissues, and bones from this fluid. Semipermeable alveoli and tubules act as valves in maintaining as much as possible the status quo, or the milieu internus.

DISTANT HISTORY (1900–1939)

By the beginning of the 20th Century, intravenous saline infusions had become commonplace, stimulated primarily by the report by Rudolph Matas on the use of infused saline solutions for the relief of acute anemia in 19 patients treated over a 3-year period in the New Orleans Charity Hospital. Although there were 12 deaths among these 19 patients, Dr. Matas reported the immediate effects of saline infusion always to be good, "with one solitary exception, in which, while the objective result was good, the subjective sensations were not satisfactory."[13]

Since 1905 there have been numerous investigations to show the depressant effects of general anesthesia upon renal function, as expressed by urine formation.[15,16,18,21,22,53,55] The dogs used as experimental animals in McNider's study received 500 ml tap water by gastric tube two hours preanesthetic. Also in this report, anuria was not reversed by the administration of solutions referred to as diuretic agents (0.9 percent sodium chloride, 20 ml per kg, or 1 percent theobromine, 1 ml per kg) if administered after a fall in systolic blood pressure and a decrease in alkali reserve.[27]

In other references to the depressant effect of ether anesthesia on renal function in the second decade of the 20th Century, there is no record of the preanesthetic preparation or of the administration of fluids, if any, during the anesthetic course.[15,16,18,21,22]

Blood transfusions with a degree of safety became possible after Landsteiner's blood groupings were described in 1900. However, for many years the procedure of transfusion was viewed with real apprehension and was employed infrequently. Prior to World War I, transfusions were administered so infrequently that, typically, one hospital bulletin (Bagley Hospital, 1910) was devoted to a full report of two transfusions occurring within the same year. In 1918, Captain Oswald H. Robertson, an American Army surgeon, found that donor blood obtained under sterile precautions and mixed with a sodium citrate solution could be preserved in an icebox for a week. Even this advance did not greatly increase the reliance on donor blood in the treatment of the war wounded. Closed systems for collecting and administering blood came into general clinical use only after World War II.

Providing a brake to what they ascribed as undue enthusiasm for saline injections, Hort and Penfold in 1911 challenged the thesis that intravenous or subcutaneous injection of large quantities of saline is an entirely innocuous procedure. These authors were critical of two basic errors of the times: "(1) The great variation in the quantities of liquid injected, together with absence of any serious attempt to graduate the volume of injection according to the body weight; (2) the wide variation in the absolute quantities of salt injected." Particular criticism was directed to the toxicity of distilled water that was allowed to stand before infusion. Neither centrifuging, filtering through cotton wool or bacterial filters, nor boiling seemed to be sufficient to prevent the fever following saline injections.[17]

Saline solutions proved a boon to physicians in the military service during World War I, particularly after a semi-closed system of administering 0.9 percent sodium chloride was devised.[25] As transfusions of blood were infrequently given, there was an effort to use colloidal solutions of gum acacia to bolster intravascular volume. With its high molecular weight, acacia was slow to pass through the capillary wall into interstitial fluid, and it exerted a definite osmotic force.[24,26,28,30] After the report in 1922 of sudden death in two patients following intravenous injections of acacia, articles on acacia seemed to drop from the literature.[31] Of course, the theory of infusing substances which would stay in the circulation was misdirected. The true dynamics of circulation involves the interstitial fluid as well as the intravascular fluid. Water passes through the capillary wall, as do all the electrolytes, urea, and glucose. During states of capillary stasis albumin, with a gram molecular weight of 69,000 and with an ellipsoidal, cigar-like shape, can pass through intercellular pores into the interstitial fluid also where it is found in concentration one-third of that in serum. Water and electrolytes return to the circulation through the venous end of the capillary wall because the oncotic pressure at that location exceeds the hydrostatic pressure. Albumin returns to the circulation through lymph channels to the thoracic duct.

Concern about the fever attendant upon or following the use of infused solutions persisted through World War II, with pyrogens being implicated and ascribed either to bacterial origin or to the chemicals inherent in the rubber infusion tubing.[32,33,35,39,48,50,56,57,59] Walter in 1946 allayed fear of the symptom complex, "intravenous reaction," by declaring and demonstrating, "There are but two fundamental requisites for a safe supply of parenteral fluids: an unlimited source of freshly distilled water, and a centralized responsibility for cleanliness in the preparation of solutions and apparatus to prevent contamination of the nonpyrogenic fluid obtained by distillation." He extolled the requirements for utmost cleanliness of the inside of the tubing and needles, removing the "bloom" from new rubber by treating it with 5 percent sodium carbonate solution in an autoclave at 250°F for 30 minutes and then rinsing with 1 percent hydrochloric acid followed by distilled water.[48]

Safety from bacterial contamination and from chemical pyrogens was not really achieved, however, until the years immediately following World War II, when hospitals slowly adopted the practice of purchasing solutions prepared under controlled conditions by pharmaceutical manufacturers who distributed the solutions in sealed disposable bottles. Disposable sterile intravenous administration sets also became available and supplanted the reusable equipment over a period of years. In the early 1950s those hospitals still making up their own solutions and reautoclaving their nondisposable infusion sets were continuing to find pyrogenic reactions among their patients.

As with other medical techniques and methods, there were ardent enthusiasts for the use of intravenous fluids, despite the reports of infection and pyrogenic reactions. Many clinicians felt that life could be sustained indefinitely with intravenous solutions of dextrose and water, or dextrose and saline, without alimentary feedings, "rendering the physician and patient absolutely independent of the gastrointestinal canal during a given period."[34]

Enthusiasm for parenteral alimentation was tempered with beliefs that the patient would develop chills if the room temperature solutions were administered too rapidly. Consequently, much effort was devoted to keeping solutions warm, with hot water bottles around the reservoir jars, or by use of hot water jackets.[38] Additional evidence of worry about cold intravenous solutions was the development of ingenious infusion sets which incorporated a mercury thermometer in the drip bulb.

Other clinicians found therapeusis to reside in the act of giving intravenous drips, because of the magical qualities of the intravenous drip itself. In 1935 JAMA carried an article of five pages extolling the value of "the drip," in which the solutions administered were never identified.[43]

Monitoring the temperature of infused solutions generated only a brief flurry of activity and was forgotten until the hazards of transfusing cold blood rapidly and/or in large volumes were implicated widely in the 1960s in causing cardiac arrhythmias.

RECENT HISTORY (1940–1950)

In the recent past, principally in the 1940s, there were many reports of specific effects of anesthesia upon renal function which caused decreased excretion of sodium in the postoperative period.[60,67,68,69] Perhaps resulting from observations of the effects of anesthesia on the kidney, there was widespread reluctance to administer salt-containing solutions, other than blood, until recent years, when it was established that the kidney responds to the functional extracellular fluid volume, a major determinant of sodium excretion.[73,84,94,96] The topic of postoperative urinary excretion of sodium is an appropriate beginning point for a discussion of recent developments.

Use of salt solutions during anesthesia and operation during the immediate post-World War II years was discouraged because of various interpretations of extensive research findings and clinical impressions of Surgery Department members at the University of Michigan Medical School, a renowned institution with an outstanding surgery faculty. Beginning in 1936, through the early months of 1950, this department issued publications dealing with postoperative salt intolerance, effects of operation and anesthesia depressing excretion of salt and water due to changes in renal function, and fluid translocations.[46,60,62,67,68,69]

To summarize pertinent conclusions from these references, there was a firm caution against giving isotonic saline solutions during the day of operation and the subsequent two postoperative days. Warnings were given concerning administration of saline solutions to hypoproteinemic, anemic, acidotic, or oliguric patients. Special recommendations were made that correction of uncompensated extracellular fluid deficiency states be made upon the basis of physiologic responses to test doses of the appropriate salt solution rather than on laboratory findings of plasma chloride, carbon dioxide combining power, NPN, plasma proteins, or the hemoglobin levels.

One of the Michigan surgery researchers was Carl A. Moyer, M.D., who had also spent a year in clinical and research activities in the Department of Anesthesiology at the Massachusetts General Hospital. In 1946 he joined the faculty of Southwestern Medical College, Dallas, Texas as Professor of Experimental Surgery. A short time later the medical school became The University of Texas Southwestern

Medical School, and Moyer became its first chairman of the Department of Surgery. Before leaving Michigan, Moyer had discredited the clinical rule, followed by the surgery department there, of giving the postoperative patient 0.5 g of salt for each 100 mg percent the plasma chloride is reported below 560 mg percent. He brought to Dallas its first experience with reports in mEq per liter ("horsepower") versus mg percent ("number of cylinders") even though laboratory determinations were still slow and laborious. A request for a serum sodium determination could take up to three days for a response, since a flame photometer was not available until the first laboratory model was delivered for the anesthesiology research laboratory in 1950. Considering the paucity of easily obtained laboratory reports, it is obvious why Moyer attracted such an avid group for his teachings of physical signs of sodium deficit, sodium excess, potassium deficit, and potassium excess as well as other evidences of acid-base derangements, later described so well in his clinical manual, *Fluid Balance*.[71]

As late as February 1950 Moyer authored an article based on data from clinical investigations at the University of Michigan.[68] In describing acute renal function changes associated with a major surgical procedure, he interpreted a clinical study to show that a salt solution is avidly retained intra- and postoperatively. Essentially this same message was conveyed by other studies.[60,62,67]

MODERN HISTORY (1950–Present)*

Over a short period in the summer of 1950, Moyer's anti-salt solution attitude underwent a change. It was altered because of postmortem findings in a series of trauma patients who underwent surgery while in states of hemorrhagic, hypovolemic shock for whom only whole blood was used as the resuscitation fluid.[70] The resultant stiff lungs, liver-lungs, or congestive atelectasis stimulated Moyer and his research associates to reproduce the findings in laboratory procedures involving anesthetized dogs, in which pulmonary red cell mass was shown to increase, while the pulmonary plasma volume decreased.

---

*Author's note: At this point in the historical review I find the narrative difficult to write without using the personal pronoun, since I was a participant in the clinical and laboratory projects with Dr. Moyer and in the clinical studies with his successors.

As a result of this combination of clinical experiences and experimental measurements, Moyer reversed his previous caveats against intraoperative administration of salt solutions, directing that a regimen for fluids be implemented to include balanced salt solutions.[70]

Within a short time we settled upon an intraoperative fluid regimen for adult patients on the elective surgical schedule, and we watched these patients carefully for signs of fluid overload or any other adverse findings. We were indeed gratified that their perioperative courses were not only acceptable, but seemed even better than patients on other operative services who did not receive balanced salt solution infusions. For the years 1950–59, our plan was to administer lactated Ringer's solution (L/R), alternating liters between plain L/R and 5 percent dextrose in L/R, 10 ml per kg body weight per hour plus L/R two times the measured blood loss, tempered with reason as influenced by urine output. Our first tempering, or moderation, came in 1959 during the investigational work by Shires and associates which resulted in the provocative article, *Changing Concept of Salt Water and Surgery.* We continued using the formula of ml per kg body weight, but only for the first two hours. In longer cases we were guided by urine output (50–100 ml per hour, or about 1 ml per kg body wt per hour) and discontinued using blood loss as a guide to a specified quantity of balanced salt solution.

It seems quite appropriate at this point to praise a remarkable man, Carl A. Moyer, M.D. (1908–1970) as a giant among physicians in an era of outstanding men and women in medicine. He was a stimulating and provocative leader of great integrity. It must not have been easy for him to reverse published opinions for which he had received considerable recognition and acclaim. His earlier influence was evident as surgeon visitors in the operating rooms at Parkland Memorial Hospital in the 1950s, mindful of Moyer and Coller's earlier admonitions, were appalled by and often complained about the volume of balanced salt solutions being administered during anesthesia and operation.

When Moyer departed Southwestern Medical School in 1952 to take the chairmanship of Surgery at Washington University in St. Louis, he left a dedicated contingent of surgeons, including Shires, and anesthesiologists who continued his clinical pursuits and laboratory investigations in fluid balance. Moyer had often expressed a sincere hope that his students' achievements would exceed his. At a conference on fluids held in Washington, D.C., in 1964, the chairman, Moyer, with obvious pride acknowledged the superior accomplishments of his former resident, G. Thomas Shires, M.D.

Based on several articles by Shires we spoke frequently of "third-space shifts" of fluids, an extrapolation from precise language not advocated by his reports. Though quite expressive, the designation "third-space shift"* is inaccurate. It does convey an understanding, however, of the functional loss of ECF from the dynamics of the circulation, sequestered as edema or translocated into muscle cells.

For example, during an intra-abdominal operation in which adequate exposure is difficult to achieve, and in which there is considerable necessary manipulation of the viscera, there may be an ECF loss equivalent to 25 to 30 percent of the preoperative volume. Such functional losses are essentially of isotonic fluid, as indicated by serum electrolyte determinations, and the losses represent internal redistribution. Part of the internal loss is into the tissue adjacent to the surgical wound in the abdominal wall, which becomes ropey, firm, and noncompressible in the immediate postoperative period, regardless of volume or type fluid administered. Additional ECF is translocated into areas where salt water tends to be sequestered as edema in response to trauma, including in this example, the splanchnic bed, mesentery, the gut wall, and even into the lumen of the bowel as ileus begins. Particularly in shock, for whatever reason it occurs, there may also be an intracellular shift of fluid with skeletal muscle cells being the major site of fluid and electrolyte sequestration.[81,82,83,89,92]

Edema of the abdominal wall (or any other surgical site) and ileus with distension of the bowel have long been recognized, but the magnitude of the loss of functional extracellular fluid has been elucidated only within the past three decades by the reports of Shires and his research and clinical associates. Another early publication of Shires and associates described the distributional changes in ECF during acute hemorrhagic shock[74] and established the rationale for fluid therapy in shock.[76,77,79,81,83]

Shires and associates have continued this work and have delineated a depression of transmembrane potential difference and an elevation of interstitial potassium in hemorrhagic shock.[89] With an

---

*There are two spaces: intracellular and extracellular. A transcellular space may be considered as a true third space, representing various collections of extracellular fluids which are not simple transudates, but which are formed by the transport activity of cells. These fluids constitute about 15 ml per kg, or 2.5 percent of total body water, and include fluids in the salivary and thyroid glands, liver, biliary tract, and respiratory mucous membrane, as well as cerebrospinal fluid and gastrointestinal secretions.

increase in interstitial potassium there is shown to be a reduction in the efficiency of an active ionic pump mechanism, or a selective increase in muscle cell permeability to sodium, related to the shock state. These latter studies utilized an ultramicroelectrode to measure directly the difference in electrical potential between the inside and outside of a muscle cell. The data suggest that muscle cells may be a principal site of fluid and electrolyte sequestration after severe, prolonged hemorrhagic shock. Only a 10 percent increase in size of muscle cells due to isotonic swelling would explain the reduction in ECF measured in hemorrhagic shock.[92]

Work continues in many laboratories and clinics on perioperative fluid administration. Future work can begin with clear evidence that there is a sequestered edema associated with the necessary manipulations in major surgical procedures, with trauma, with significant blood loss, and with shock.

EPILOGUE

No single regimen for fluid administration will apply to patients with varying physical status and disease processes and scheduled for a variety of operations. We acknowledge the obvious fact that throughout the world, differing routines for intraoperative fluids are followed. These routines may range from no fluids at all, to blood only, and some may include albumin or mannitol on a definitely timed basis. Under any regimen, it seems that a majority of patients survive, some because of fluid administration and others despite it.

As a central theme of our precepts we feel that homeostatic mechanisms in the anesthetized patient are best maintained if fluid administration helps to preserve normal renal function while replacing ECF translocated from the dynamic pool. Our regimen, therefore, is strongly influenced by recent developments in the history of sequestered edema.[94]

A. We begin with 5 percent dextrose in water (D5W) up to 500 ml, and continue with 5 percent dextrose in balanced salt solutions (D5BS) in the following procedures:

(1) *Intra-abdominal and hip operations.* 12 to 15 ml per kg body weight during the first hour, and 6 to 10 ml per kg per hour for the next two hours, varied as indicated by the degree of surgical manipulation (trauma), arterial pressure, pulse, urine output and, in certain cases, central venous pressure or pulmonary wedge

pressure. For operations beyond three hours, we continue with a balanced salt solution without glucose at a rate to assure urinary output of 50 to 100 ml per hour.

(2) *Intrathoracic (noncardiac) operations.* 6 to 10 ml per kg per hour.

(3) *Extremities and major superficial operations.* 6 to 10 ml per kg per hour varied after the first hour as indicated by degree of operative manipulation (trauma), arterial pressure, and pulse.

B. We begin and continue with D5BS in these operations:

(1) *Intracranial procedures.* Balanced salt solutions are administered only in volumes sufficient to keep the venous channel (IV) open until the surgeon begins the closure; then begin replacement with balanced salt solutions as indicated by urine output.

(2) *Transurethral prostatic surgery.* 3 to 6 ml per kg per hour while watching volume by operative "washwater" absorbed through the prostatic bed.

C. We begin and continue with D5W in volumes sufficient to keep the IV open (i.e., minimal fluids where operative trauma is limited) in these procedures:

(1) *Microsurgery of the ear and larynx.*

(2) *Most ophthalmic operations.*

D. We limit the total dextrose administered to a maximum of 125g.

E. We transfuse with whole blood or its equivalent in blood component therapy when blood loss exceeds 20 percent of estimated blood volume.

F. We monitor urine output on all major trauma operations and all predicted to be lengthy procedures.

HISTORICAL REFERENCES LISTED CHRONOLOGICALLY

Numbers in parentheses indicate references for recommended reading not specifically discussed in this article, although they relate to the state of the art at that time in history.

1. HARVEY, WILLIAM: *Exercitatio anatomica de motu cordis et sanguinis,* 1628. Quoted in *The Works of William Harvey,* London, the Sydenham Society, 1847.
(Translated by Robert Willis, a country practitioner commissioned by the Sydenham Society to investigate and compare the 1653 English translation to the original Latin treatise of 1628. He rejected the 1653

version and conducted an original translation of Harvey's dissertation on the circulation of the blood.)

2. HARVEY, WILLIAM: *Exercitatio anatomica de motu cordis et sanguinus in animalibus.* The Classics of Medicine Library, Birmingham, 1978.
(A facsimile of the 1628 Francofurti edition together with the Keynes English translation of 1928.)

3. BISHOP SPRATT: In *History of the Royal Society of London,* 1667, p 317.
(The first recorded injection of drugs into veins, opium and crocus mettallorum into dogs through a quill attached to a small bladder, by Sir Christopher Wren.)

4. ELSHOLTZ, JS: Quoted in *The Lure of Medical History,* as translated by Ethel Gladstone.

Chap I: Calif and West Med 38:432, 1933.

CLYSMATICA NOVA

*"Ratio, qua in venam fectam
Editio Secunda,
Varijs experimentis per Germanium,
Angliam, Gallias atque Italiam factis,
nec non Iconibus aliquor illustrata*

"If a tankard of wine is poured into a river, the wine, together with the water, flows into the sea. In just the same way whatever liquid is injected into a vein must necessarily reach the heart, together with the circulating blood."   1661

Chap III: Calif and West Med 39:45, 1933.

THE NEW CLYSTER
or
THE ART OF THE ENEMA

applied to arteries and veins by injection through a syringe.

Chaps V and VII: Calif and West Med 39:119, 1933.

Simple and reciprocal transfusions in animals; IV injections of opium, carthartics, emetics, and arsenic to dogs; liquor balsamici, aqua plantagiuis, aqua cardnibenedicti, and aqua cochleariae to men.

[Syringe and needles are used and referred to!]

Chap IX and XII: Calif and West Med 39:190, 1933.

CLYSMATICA NOVA
Johann Sig. Elshorst

Contains references to work of the French who transfused blood of a lamb into a man; of the British who treated patients by bleeding them; and to work of the Italians and Germans, "... let the Italians contend with the French about their priority, and the English with the Germans," but ... "ambition does not trouble me greatly, so that I would grudge a bit of fame to others," and further, "I first combined these experiments properly."   1667

5. O'Shaughnessy, WB: *Proposal of a new method of treating the blue epidemic cholera by the injection of highly-oxygenized salts into the venous system.* Lancet 1:366, 1831–32.
(In cholera a large proportion of water is lost, neutral saline ingredients are lost, free alkali disappears, urine is suppressed and urea increases, and globular structure of blood is unchanged, as described by the author.)

6. Lewins, R: Letter to the editor. Lancet 2:243, 1831–32.
(Injection of saline solutions in extraordinary quantities into the veins of patients having malignant cholera.)

7. Latta, T: Letter to the editor. Lancet 2:274, 1831–32.
(Documents communicated by the Central Board of Health, London, relative to the treatment of cholera by the copious injection of aqueous and saline fluids into the veins.)

(8.) O'Shaughnessy, WB: *Chemical pathology of cholera.* Lancet 2:225, 1831–32.
(An eight-page diatribe against another physician who disagrees with the author on the chemical pathology of malignant cholera.)

9. Hunter, C: *Practical remarks on the hypodermical treatment of disease.* Lancet 2:444, 675, 1863.
(Frequent sepsis occurred but it was not ascribed to hypodermic technique on injections. This was pre-Listerian.)

10. Fagge, CH: *A case of diabetic coma treated with partial success by the injection of a saline solution into the blood.* Guy's Hosp Rep 19:173, 1874.
(The earlier observations made on cholera stimulated fluid administration in the treatment of diabetic coma where, for the first time, dehydration was described as a feature of this state.)

11. LISTER, JOSEPH: *A contribution to the germ theory of putrefaction and other fermentative changes, and to the natural history of torulae and bacteria.* Trans Royal Soc Edinburgh 27, T–2, 1875.
    ("It is well known that organic substances, when left exposed under ordinary circumstances, undergo alterations in their qualities. For example, an infusion of malt experiences the alcoholic fermentation; a basin of paste prepared from wheaten flour becomes mouldy; or, again, a piece of meat putrefies when so treated. The microscope shows that each of these changes is attended by the development of minute organisms . . . characterized by astonishing powers of locomotion, and, from their rod-like form, termed *Bacteria.*
    "The Germ Theory supposes that the organisms are the causes of the changes; that the germs of these minute living things, diffusible in proportion to their minuteness, are omnipresent in the world around us, and are sure to gain access to any exposed organic substance; and, having thus reached it, develop if it prove a favourable *nidus,* and by their growth determine the chemical changes; and further, that these organisms, minute though they appear to us, form no exception to the general law of living beings, that they originate from similar beings by parentage.")

12. BERNARD, CLAUDE: *Le cons sur les phenomenes de la vie communs aux animaux et aux vegetaux.* Balliere, Paris, 1879.
    (More than a century ago, Bernard, a giant among nineteenth century physiologists, wrote of "that bit of primeval sea within us"—the milieu internus or the internal environment, the true medium in which we live, so isolated from the world that atmospheric disturbances cannot alter it or penetrate beyond it.)

13. MATAS, RUDOLPH: *A clinical report on intravenous saline infusion in the wards of the New Orleans Charity Hospital, from June 1888 to June 1891.* New Orleans Med Surg J. 19:1, 1891.
    (First historical attempt to infuse saline solution for the relief of acute anemia. "Good results" in patients treated for shock, hemorrhage, or exhaustion.)

14. FORTESQUE-BRICKDALE,F: *A contribution to the history of intravenous injection of drugs.* Guy's Hosp Rep 58:15, 1904.
    (Ascribed to Muratori in the Rer. Ital. Script., t iii, pars. ii, p. 1241, the earliest recorded administration of blood was in 1492 given to Pope Innocent VIII who died, as did the three boys who were used as donors. The next allusion to blood transfusions was by DeColle, Ars parendi medicamente, Cap.vii, p. 170, Venet. 1628.)

15. PRINGLE, H, MAUNSELL, RCB, AND PRINGLE, S: *Clinical effects of ether anaesthesia on renal activity.* Br Med J 2:542, 1905.
    (Oliguria, sodium and nitrogen excretion diminished. No recording of intraoperative fluids administered, if any.)

16. HAWK, PB: *Urine formation during ether anesthesia.* Arch Intern Med 8:177, 1911.
    (Oliguria and elevation of non-protein nitrogen. No recording of intraoperative fluids administered.)

17. HORT, EC AND PENFOLD, WJ: *The dangers of saline injections.* Br Med J 2:1589, 1911.
    ("In recent years the practice of injecting hot solutions of saline into a vein, or under the skin, has greatly increased. . . . The undesirable effects that we encountered include fever, rigors, subnormal temperatures, diarrhoea, intestinal haemorrhage, Cheyne-Stokes breathing, convulsions, and sudden death. The last two we have only met with after injection of strongly hypertonic solutions. . . . The grave sequel to large saline injections (in man) of pulmonary oedema has recently been noted. To this list of clinical drawbacks to saline injections in animals may be added the onset of glycosuria. We must also note the histological changes observed by other workers on this subject. Raum (1892), for example, showed that intravenous injection of the dog with normal saline was followed by vacuolation of the liver cells. Allbrecht (1907) found that the red cells of animals were damaged by large injections of normal saline; Rossle (1907) observed degenerative changes in the heart muscle and capillary walls of animals similarly injected, and Hossli found that saline injections caused in animals fatty changes in the heart muscle and kidneys. . . .

    "In a recent paper by Wechselmann (1911), attention is called to the dangers of intravenous injection of saline solutions of salvarsan. This observer believes that many of the unpleasant effects which he found to follow the injection of salvarsan were directly due to bacteria he found in the distilled water of the solutions he injected. . . .

    "We are driven to the suggestion that the fever which always follows the injection of suitable quantities of distilled water allowed to stand is caused by soluble products, perhaps of bacterial origin, and is not directly due to bacteria as such or to unaltered protein.")

18. MILLER, RH AND CABOT, H: *The effect of anesthesia and operation on the kidney function, as shown by the phenosulphonephthalein test.* Arch Intern Med 15:369, 1915.
    (PSP excretion diminished 20 percent. No recording of intraoperative fluids administered.)

19. HOLT, E, COURTNEY, A, AND FALES, HL: *The chemical composition of diarrheal as compared with normal stools in infants.* Am J Dis Child 9:213, 1915.
    (As noted by Moyer (71), "It was recognized that another deadly disease, infantile diarrhea, had many of the features of cholera. With their studies of this complex, Holt, Courtney, and Fales, and Howland and Marriott* so stirred the interest of pediatricians in body fluids that

they have been preeminent in this subject ever since. The fundamental contributions of Gamble, Hartmann and Darrow bear witness to this. The fundamental physical and chemical discoveries of Gibbs, Henderson, Van Slyke, Hastings, Gamble, and Peters are the foundations for the development of fluid therapy. Links between the physical chemists, biochemists and clinicians are gradually being made."
[*See next reference, #20.])

20. HOWLAND, J AND MARRIOTT, WM: *Acidosis occurring with diarrhea.* Am J Dis Child 11:309, 1916.

21. MACNIDER, W DE B: *A pathological study of the naturally acquired chronic nephropathy of the dog, Part I.* J Med Research 34:177, 1916. (See ref #27.)

22. MACNIDER, W DE B: *A pathological and physiological study of the naturally nephropathic kidney of the dog, rendered acutely nephropathic by uranium or by an anesthetic, Part II.* J Med Research 34:199, 1916. (See ref. 27.)

23. MACHT, DI: *The history of intravenous and subcutaneous administration of drugs.* JAMA 66:856, 1916.
(An inquiry into the historical development of the administration of substances by subcutaneous or intravenous injection. Of special interest are the four references to publications on intravenous air embolism written between 1773 and 1823.)

24. HURWITZ, SH: *Intravenous injections of colloidal solutions of acacia in hemorrhage.* JAMA 68:699, 1917.
("By virtue of its colloidal nature, blood exerts a mechanical effect in raising the blood pressure by filling the vascular system with a slowly diffusible fluid . . . the use of saline solution is not as efficacious as whole blood in the treatment of hemorrhage . . . the conclusion is justified that fluid introduced in colloidal combination leaves the vascular system more slowly than 'free' fluid . . . intravenous injections of colloidal gelatin solutions are not diuretic, and their introduction into the circulating stream results in a higher and in a more sustained blood pressure . . . than saline . . . suggested to us the use of an acacia-Locke solution therapeutically in man and in animals for the purpose of combating the immediate mechanical ill effects of lowered pressure following excessive hemorrhage . . . gum acacia is an acid of high molecular weight, composed of an acid nucleus to which are attached a number of different carbohydrate radicals.")

25. FIASCHI, P: *The administration of saline solutions.* (New Inventions.) Lancet 2:794, 1917.
(A semiclosed system of administering 0.9 percent NaCl in glass-distilled water is described for ease of use in the military service.)

26. CANNON, WB: *Traumatic shock.* War Medicine 2:1367, 1919.
("In the absence of blood, use Bayliss gum-salt solution, which raises pressure by increasing volume and thereby causes more rapid circulation and better employment of the corpuscles as oxygen carriers.")

27. MACNIDER, W DE B: *A study of anurias occurring in normal animals during the use of general anesthetics.* J Pharmacol Exp Ther 15:249, 1920.
(43 of 131 dogs became anuric during the course of anesthesia produced either by di-ethyl ether, chloroform, or "Grehant's anesthetic . . . mixture which consists of chloroform, alcohol, and water by stomach tube. . . ." The anesthetic technique was not defined, nor was there a statement about ventilation or adequacy of the airway of the experimental animals. Anuria occurred consistently when the blood pressure fell and when the alkali reserve was reduced. The anuria was not reversed by the administration of solutions referred to as diuretic agents, either 0.9 percent sodium chloride (20 ml per kg body wt) or 1 percent theobromine (1 ml per kg body wt). There was surgical manipulation in opening the abdomen and implanting catheters in the ureters of these experimental animals.)

28. WHITE, HL AND ERLANGER, J: *The effect on the composition of the blood of maintaining an increased blood volume by the intravenous injection of a hypertonic solution of gum acacia and glucose in normal, asphyxiated and shocked dogs.* Am J Physiol 54:1, 1920.
(Increase in blood volume; questionable increase in plasma proteins; gum acacia seems to hold water in circulation; marked hyperglycemia; crystalloid osmotic pressure is inconstant.)

(29.) ROGERS, L: *The mortality and prognosis of cholera treated by the author's hypertonic saline method, based on 2000 cases.* Lancet 1:1079, 1921.
(This author was impressed with the need for noncolloid intravenous solutions to reduce the hematocrit of 70 often found in cholera. With hypertonic saline he reduced the death rate from 59 percent to 32 percent of cholera patients. The inventory is not clear, however.)

30. BAYLISS, WM: *The action of gum acacia on the circulation.* J Pharmacol Exp Ther 15:29, 1920–21.
(7 percent gum acacia in 0.9 percent sodium chloride was used in experimental animals to replace up to 75 percent blood volume loss. Urine volume was depressed. Survival rates were not clearly defined.)

31. LEE, RV: *Sudden death in two patients following intravenous injections of acacia.* JAMA 79:9, 1922.
("Results . . . give the impression that this agent is not entirely harm-

less ... the dangers of intravenous medication [of any kind] are emphasized again, and these are not confined to acacia...." This closed the fifth year of articles on the salubrious effects of gum acacia. The subject seemed to drop from the literature after 1922.)

32. SEIBERT, FB: *Fever-producing substance found in some distilled waters.* Am J Physiol 67:90, 1923.
("Emphasis must again be placed upon the fact that distilled water kept under ordinary conditions is not necessarily as pure and as physiologically harmless as is usually supposed ... it can be seen that one is not able in any hospital or research laboratory to take for granted that a physiological saline made by dissolving C.P. salt in distilled water taken from a tank and then autoclaving, is physiologically inert ... a pyrogenic substance ... develops on standing, is filterable, and is of bacterial origin.")

33. EGGLESTON, C, ET AL: *The status of intravenous therapy.* JAMA 88:1798, 1927.
(This is a report by the special committee appointed by the Therapeutic Research Committee of the Council on Pharmacy and Chemistry of the AMA. The committee recognized the value of intravenous therapy and urged its use under appropriate conditions, emphasizing the fact that the injection of any foreign substance directly into the human bloodstream is a serious undertaking. A concern was expressed about the growing tendency on the part of many physicians to resort to intravenous injections under conditions in which it is of dubious value if not potentially harmful. Indications for intravenous therapy included emergency measures, such as in the treatment of shock, toxemia, and hemorrhage. Other indications included the use of intravenous medication which is indicated when greater intensity of action is required than can be secured by other methods, and when the volume of the dose is too large to be given by intramuscular injection. The committee recognized also their indications to secure direct action of the infused chemicals within the bloodstream. Intravenous therapy was deemed contraindicated in the absence of specific indications. Most of the contraindications centered around sterility of the solutions being introduced and the possible decomposition of injectables in the process of sterilization. This committee was particularly concerned with pyrogenic substances not removed by either distillation or by heat sterilization. Judging by the committee's admonitions, there must have been a great number of complications occurring subsequent to intravenous infusions.)

34. HENDON, GA: *Venoclysis.* JAMA 95:1175, 1930.
("A patient weighing 150 pounds can easily assimilate two pounds of dextrose a day. My experience indicates that no patient need ever die of dehydration or starvation alone: that not only life but a fair

degree of physical prosperity can be sustained over a period of at least sixteen days without alimentary feeding: that venoclysis renders the physician and patient absolutely independent of the gastrointestinal canal during a given period. . . . Venoclysis furnishes a method by which nutrition can be supported independent of the alimentary canal, dehydration prevented, acidosis overcome, infection combatted, and toxins diluted to a degree of innocuous attenuation." This author performed all of his venoclyses by cutting down upon and suturing into the veins a silver or a gold-plated cannula of a 12-gauge diameter. This author was interested in glucose tolerance curves obtained by the infusion of 10 percent dextrose solution. This article was written at a time when considerable debate was in progress over the merits of dextrose in water as compared with isotonic saline solutions for intravenous injections.)

35. GALLIE, WE AND HARRIS, RI: *The continuous intravenous administration of physiological salt solution.* Ann Surg 91:422, 1930.

(These authors were taking the opposite view of that expressed in ref #34, that is, this report concerned the use of intravenous saline solutions without dextrose. Specific recommendations were made that the vein chosen should be just large enough to accommodate the cannula, "Since the smaller the vein the faster will be the rate of flow through it for any given rate of administration. This minimizes the danger of clotting." The authors were particularly concerned with the sterility of solutions and presented a diagram of the Pyrex bottle utilized to sterilize solutions, with a Murphy drip bulb attached to an outlet tube fused in the side of the flask. Among the discussants of the paper was Dr. Alexis Carrel, later noted for his work in tissue cultures. He remarked that during World War I he devised a roller pump to drive fluid into veins. His electrically driven roller pump apparently was the predecessor of the roller pump used many years later in an extracorporeal oxygenator system.)

(36.) HORSLEY, JS AND HORSLEY, GW: *Continuous intravenous injection of dextrose in Ringer's solution: Its technic and indications, and a new intravenous cannula.* Arch Surg 22:86, 1931.

(An intravenous technic adopted by the authors only because dextrose could not be given by proctoclysis!)

(37.) BEARD, JW AND BLALOCK, A: *Intravenous injections: A study of the composition of the blood during continuous trauma to the intestines when no fluid is injected and when fluid is injected continuously.* J Clin Invest 2:249, 1932.

(Using a standardized model of the deeply anesthetized dog sustaining trauma to the intestines until a state of shock was produced, these authors studied the fluid exuding from the intestines and treated the generalized shock status with a variety of solutions. Despite noting the increasing hemoconcentration of the blood, they did not inject crystalloid solutions in volumes sufficient to restore an acceptable blood pressure. Instead, they expressed the belief that the rapid loss of solutions of crystalloids from the bloodstream explained the transitory beneficial effects of such injections but did not explain why the condition of the patient should often be worse after fluid administration. The authors seemed to form definite opinions against the use of crystalloid solutions despite the distinct impression that the blood pressure climbed more rapidly after the injection of crystalloid solutions was stopped than in an animal in a similar shocked condition in which no fluids had been introduced. They did note that gum acacia solutions seemed to have an advantage over solutions of crystalloids, and that they were associated with an immediate increase in plasma volume, even though the protein content of the serum was decreased. Despite this favorable report on acacia, the authors did not pursue experimental work with it, nor did they entertain the thought that acacia would be indicated.)

38. THEODORE, S: *Improved method for maintaining uniformity of temperature of infusions.* Hosp Prog 1933.

(In the early 1930s great concern was expressed over the high incidence of chills and fever accompanying the infusion of intravenous drugs. These reactions were sometimes ascribed to pyrogens in the fluids and at other times to the body's response to receiving cold, or at least nonwarmed, solutions. This article describes a cylindrical jacket of heavy steel of the exact diameter to accommodate a Kelley bottle, an open-top intravenous infusion bottle. This jacket contained a thermometer and had a circular lid which could be opened for refilling the cylinder when the water inside cooled sufficiently. As described, this radiator would require refilling with hot water, or warm water, only five times for a six-hour infusion. This technic supplanted the older method of refilling two hot water bottles every 15 minutes and placing them around the infusion bottle. For a six-hour infusion, this would mean a total of 48 hot water bottles to be refilled. This labor-saving device was recommended also to keep bottles of donor blood warm while the contents were being infused.)

39. RADEMAKER, L: *Reactions after intravenous infusions.* Surg Gynecol Obstet 56:956, 1933.

(The author described a system of strict control of intravenous solutions from the time they are distilled to the types bottles in which the distillate is captured to the preparation of the rubber infusion tubing by filling the tubing with 10 percent sodium hydroxide for 12–24 hours, washing in running water for two hours, and boiling in distilled water for one-half hour before using. Preparing the solutions in a central room by graduate nurses reportedly reduced adverse reactions from 30 percent to 0.1 percent of patients receiving intravenous fluid administrations. This low incidence of reactions is somewhat surprising, since the preparation of fluids was still not a completely sterile process. " . . . Strict rules were developed for cleansing of all glassware. The flasks and graduates are first washed in tincture of green soap and hot water and rinsed in tap water. The standard cleaning solution of potassium bichromate and sulfuric acid is then used. The glassware is next rinsed four times with tap water and six times with freshly distilled water. It is then ready for use.")

(40.) HYMAN, HT AND HIRSCHFELD, S: *The therapeutics of the intravenous drip.* JAMA 100:305, 1933.
("The vehicle to be introduced in the drip is a matter of secondary importance.")

(41.) JONES, CM AND EATON, FB: *Postoperative nutritional edema.* Arch Surg 27:159, 1933.

(42.) SCHATZ, WJ: *How old is the syringe in parenteral procedure?* Clinical Excerpts 8(5):1, 1934.

43. HYMAN, HT AND TOUROFF, ASW: *Therapeutics of the intravenous drip: Further observations.* JAMA 104:446, 1935.
(Five pages extolling the value of "the drip" without mentioning the solution. Compare the term, drip, with venoclysis and phleboclysis.)

(44.) WARTHEN, HJ: *Massive intravenous injections: An experimental study.* Arch Surg 30:199, 1935.

(45.) COLLER, FA: *Dehydration* (an editorial). Surg Gynecol Obstet 63:249, 1936.

46. COLLER, FA, DICK, VS, AND MADDOCK, WG: *Maintenance of normal water exchange with intravenous fluids.* JAMA 107:1522, 1936.

(47.) MASON, JT: *Practical considerations, in shock, dehydration, starvation, etc.* Industrial Medicine 5:16, 1936.

48. WALTER, CW: *Preparation of safe intravenous solutions.* Surg Gynecol Obstet 63:643, 1936.

49. GAMBLE, JL: *Extracellular fluid and its vicissitudes.* Bull Johns Hopkins Hosp 61:151, 1937.
(Beautifully written text on extracellular fluid and its condiments. It lacks the concept of a mobile pool. It provides an excellent anatomic description of the extracellular fluid as a force, largely stationary, lending stability to physico-chemical conditions within the organism.)

50. BLEYER, LF AND ROHDE, M: *A method for producing pyrogen-free water for intravenous therapy.* Am J Surg 37:136, 1937.

(51.) PORTER, HB: *Intravenous drip: Review of the literature and technique of this method of fluid administration.* Military Surgeon 2:192 March, 1937.

(52.) HABEIN, HC: *The intravenous use of fluids.* In *Collected Papers of the Mayo Clinic & Mayo Foundation,* Vol 30, p 963, 1938.

53. STEWART, JD AND ROURKE, GM: *Changes in blood and interstitial fluid resulting from surgical operation and ether anesthesia.* J Clin Invest 17:413, 1938.
(Inhibition of water diuresis intraoperatively and postoperatively despite sufficient 5 percent D/W to lower sodium by 26 mEq per liter and chloride by 18.5 mEq per liter!! Reduction in plasma volume may be greater than accounted for by hemorrhage.)

(54.) WINSLOW, SB: *Dextrose utilization in surgical patients.* Surgery 4:867, 1938.
("It protects the liver and avoids the edema which may result from the promiscuous use of physiologic solution of sodium chloride.")

55. SMITH, HW, ET AL: *Effects of spinal anesthesia on circulation in normal, unoperated man with reference to autonomy of arterioles, and especially those of renal circulation.* J Clin Invest 18:319, 1939.

56. HARTMAN, FW: *The elimination of rubber tubing on intravenous sets.* Ann Surg 111:498, 1940.

57. TOVELL, RM AND PATTERSON, RL: *Intravenous therapy: A hospital problem for which the anesthetist may provide a solution.* Anesth Analg 19:171, 1940.

(58.) KEELEY, JL: *Intravenous injections and infusions.* Am J Surg 50:485, 1940.

59. WALTER, CW: *The relation of proper preparation of solutions for intravenous therapy to febrile reactions.* Ann Surg 112:603, 1940.
(Equipment problems: origin of hypodermic medication was pre-Listerian (1850s); early IV sets without drip bulbs (1880–1920); pyrogens in distilled water (1930s); preparation of rubber IV tubing (1930s); the relation of proper preparation of solutions for intravenous therapy to febrile reactions.)

60. COLLER, FA, ET AL: *Postoperative salt intolerance.* Ann Surg 119:533, 1944.
("There is a high incidence of 'salt intolerance' following general anesthesia; . . . give no isotonic saline or Ringer's solution on operative day and following two days; . . . treat fluid deficiency states on responses to test doses rather than on measured electrolytes." In the recent past this was perhaps the most significant article in influencing fluid administration during anesthesia and operation, proscribing the use of salt solutions. It reports a very sophisticated clinical study of urinary sodium excretion by a series of patients undergoing the same operation, combined abdominoperineal excision of the rectum for carcinoma. (The Miles' operation, devised by British surgeon William E. Miles, 1869–1947.) These patients were prepared for operation by

the Miles' regimen of purging with magnesium sulfate followed by cleansing soap suds enemas. Then they received 125 ml 0.9 percent sodium chloride per hour for four hours during the anesthesia and operation. In studying urinary output no sodium was found.

Conclusions then were that under circumstances of anesthesia and operation there is either a renal intolerance to salt or a renal inability to excrete salt during an operation. Conclusions today would be that an adult patient prepared by the Miles' regimen would have the extracellular fluid volume diminished by two to four liters which would be significantly further reduced by translocation accompanying the necessary trauma of such an extensive surgical procedure. Consequently, today the absence of sodium in the urine would be interpreted as the normal action of the kidney in protecting a reduced extracellular fluid volume.)

(61.) MOYER, CA, ET AL: *A study of the interrelationship of salt solutions, serum and defibrinated blood in the treatment of severely scalded, anesthetized dogs.* Ann Surg 120:367, 1944.

62. COLLER, FA, ET AL: *Translocation of fluid produced by the intravenous administration of isotonic salt solutions in man postoperatively.* Ann Surg 122:663, 1945.
(Postoperative injection of 0.9 percent sodium chloride results in its being retained, more than 50 percent. Hypotonic solutions are retained also, although extra free water is provided for elimination by skin and lungs. Translocations, if any, are not explained.)

(63.) WOLF, AV: *Retention and excretion of continuously administered salt solutions.* Am J Physiol 143:572, 1945.

(64.) HOLMES, JH AND PAINTER, EE: *The role of the extracellular fluid in traumatic shock in dogs.* Am J Physiol 148:201, 1947.
(ECF volume unchanged in shock due to muscle trauma. ECF is transferred from uninjured areas to the blood, thence to traumatized area. IV 0.9 percent sodium chloride enters injured area.)

65. HOWARD-JONES, N: *A critical study of the origins and early development of hypodermic medication.* J Hist Med 2:201, 1947.
(Who invented the hypodermic syringe?
—— Not Rynd of Ireland (retractable trocar, 1845).
—— Not Wood of Scotland (graduated syringe, 1843 or 1853, or 1858).
—— Not Pravaz of France (trocar and cannula, 1845).
—— Not Luer of France (eliminated the screw piston, 1860).
There was no such invention as the syringe. It just happened!)

(66.) MOYER, CA, LEVIN, M, AND KLINGE, FW: *The volume and composition of parenteral fluids and clinical problems of body fluid equilibrium.* South Med J 40:479, 1947.

67. MOYER, CA, ET AL: *Some effects of an operation, anesthesia and composition of parenteral fluids upon the excretion of water and salt.* South Surg 15:218, 1949.
(Volatile general anesthetic agents depress renal excretion. Depressed excretion of water, sodium, and chloride given in postoperative period. "Pre-renal deviation of fluid into injured area can scarcely be responsible.")

68. MOYER, CA: *Acute temporary changes in renal function associated with major surgical procedures.* Surgery 27:198, 1950.
(Salt solution is avidly retained during and after operation (combined A-P resection). "Fundamental causes for changes in renal function during operations are still unknown." Secretion of ECF into injured areas might change renal function. There may be some distributional shift.)

(69.) JOHNSON, HT, ET AL: *Postoperative salt retention and its relation to increased adrenal cortical function.* Ann Surg 132:374, 1950.

70. JENKINS, MT, ET AL: *Congestive atelectasis—A complication of the intravenous infusion of fluids.* Ann Surg 132:3, 1950.
(Red cell mass in lungs increased; plasma volume in lungs decreased. Turning point in authors' attitudes leading to advocacy of infusing salt solutions intraoperatively.)
(Authors' intraoperative fluid regimen, 1950–59: Lactated Ringer's solution, alternating with 5 percent dextrose in L/R, 10 ml per kg body wt per hour; plus L/R equivalent to 2× blood loss, tempered with reason as influenced by urine output.)

71. MOYER, CA: *Fluid Balance: A Clinical Manual.* Year Book Publishers, Chicago, 1952.
(Written before clinical electrolyte determinations became easily and rapidly obtainable, this little volume was and is a goldmine of clinical signs. Particularly well described are disturbances in body fluid equilibrium: in volume, in electrolytic osmolar concentration, in composition, in distribution, and, less well described, in rate of internal exchange.)

(72.) DECOSSE, JJ, ET AL: *The mechanism of hyponatremia and hypotonicity after surgical trauma.* Surgery 40:27, 1956.
(Postoperative hyponatremia and hypochloremia. Expanded ECF? Is there really an ECF? Intraoperative fluids not recorded.)

73. SHIRES, GT, WILLIAMS, J, AND BROWN, F: *Changing concept of salt water and surgery.* Texas J Med 55:1, 1959.
(Sequestration of ECF during operations (third-space shift); reduced functional extracellular fluid; diminished renal sodium excretion. This article introduced the modern concept of fluid translocation due to trauma and/or shock.)

74. SHIRES, GT, ET AL: *Distributional changes in extracellular fluid during acute hemorrhagic shock.* Surg Forum 11:115, 1960.
(Triple isotope technic for simultaneous measurement of red blood cell mass (^{51}Cr), plasma volume (^{131}I tagged serum albumin), ECF volume (^{35}S labeled Na_2SO_4). Demonstrated loss of functional ECF after hemorrhage.)

(75.) WOLFMAN, EF, ET AL: *Donor blood and isotonic salt solution.* Arch Surg 86:869, 1963.

76. SHIRES, GT, CARRICO, CJ, AND COLN, D: *The role of the extracellular fluid in shock.* Int Anesth Clin 2:435, 1964.
(Blood loss alone if sufficiently large also results in losses of ECF from the dynamics of the circulation.)

77. SHIRES, GT, ET AL: *Fluid therapy in hemorrhagic shock.* Arch Surg 88:688, 1964.
(Demonstrated the ECF to be a very mobile huge pool of water, electrolytes, and metabolic components. Showed a disparate reduction of functional ECF in hemorrhagic shock, indicating intraoperative administration of balanced salt solutions as an adjunct to blood replacement.)

(78.) FAULCONER, A, JR., AND KEYS, TE: *Accessory agencies and technics.* In *Foundations of Anesthesiology, Vol II.* Charles C Thomas, Springfield, Illinois, 1965.

79. JENKINS, MT, GIESECKE, AH, AND SHIRES, GT: *Electrolyte therapy in shock: Management during anesthesia.* In ORKIN, LR (ED): *Clinical Management of the Patient in Shock.* Clinical Anesthesia Series, Vol 2, FA Davis, Philadelphia, 1965, p 39.

(80.) SLONIM, M AND STAHL, WM, JR: *Sodium and water content of connective versus cellular tissue following hemorrhage.* Surg Forum 19:53, 1968.

81. SHIRES, GT AND CARRICO, CJ: *Current status of the shock problem.* Curr. Probl. Surg., monograph, Year Book Medical Publishers, Chicago, 1966.
(Fluid distribution changes in hemorrhagic shock: "... an isotonic internal redistribution or translocation of extracellular fluid into the intracellular compartment.... Direct evidence ... that skeletal muscle cells undergo isotonic swelling...."

82. GROSSMAN, R: *Intracellular potentials of motor cortex neurons in cerebral ischemia.* Electroencephalogr Clin Neurophysiol 24:291, 1968.
(Fluid and electrolyte sequestration in the intracellular mass of neurons in the brain in response to hemorrhagic shock.)

83. JENKINS, MT AND GIESECKE, AH: *Anesthesia considerations.* In SHIRES,

GT (ED): *Care of the Trauma Patient.* McGraw-Hill, New York, 1966, p 82.
84. JENKINS, MT AND GIESECKE, AH: *Clinical questions related to fluids.* In JENKINS, MT (ED): *Common and Uncommon Problems in Anesthesiology.* Clinical Anesthesia Series, Vol 3, FA Davis, Philadelphia, 1968, p 211.
85. SHIRES, GT, ET AL: *Principles in treatment of severely injured patients: The management of anesthesia for trauma.* WELCH, CE:In *Advances in Surgery, Vol 4,* Year Book Medical Publishers, Chicago, 1970, p 289.
(86.) JENKINS, MT: *Complications in fluid therapy.* In SAIDMAN, L AND MOYA, F (EDS): *Complications of Anesthesia.* Charles C Thomas, Springfield, Illinois, 1970, p 124.
(87.) JENKINS, MT: *Problems due to endocrine disorders.* In SAIDMAN L AND MOYA, F (EDS): *Complications in anesthesia.* Charles C Thomas, Springfield, Illinois, 1970, p 252.
(88.) JENKINS, MT: *ADH, water, and salt.* In *Proceedings of the Third Asian-Australasian Congress on Anaesthesia.* Butterworths, Australia, 1970, p 59.
89. CUNNINGHAM, JN, JR, SHIRES, GT, AND WAGNER, Y: *Cellular transport defects in hemorrhagic shock.* Surgery 70:215, 1971.
(In hemorrhagic shock there is a depression of transmembrane potential difference and an elevation of interstitial potassium—a reduction in the efficiency of an active ionic pump mechanism or a selective increase in muscle cell permeability to sodium.)
(90.) CUNNINGHAM, JN, JR, SHIRES, GT, AND WAGNER, Y: *Changes in intracellular sodium and potassium content of red blood cells in trauma and shock.* Am J Surg 122:650, 1971.
(Severe hemorrhagic shock of significant duration is associated with elevation of internal sodium concentration in red cells—part of a process involving a generalized change in cellular composition and function in hemorrhagic shock.)
(91.) SHIRES, GT, ET AL: *Alterations in cellular membrane function during hemorrhagic shock in primates.* Ann Surg 176:288, 1972.
(Marked decrease in both total extracellular water and muscle extracellular water. Significant increase in intracellular sodium concentration with prolonged muscle membrane depolarization.)
92. SHIRES, GT, CARRICO, CJ, AND CANIZARO, PC: *Shock.* In DUNPHY, JE (ED): *Major Problems in Clinical Surgery,* Vol XIII. WB Saunders, Philadelphia, 1973.
(A compilation of the major problems associated with severe bodily injury, their consequences, and rational approaches to treatment. This includes a study of the effects of shock on cellular function and

the translocation of fluids from the extracellular to the intracellular compartments.)

(93.) JENKINS, MT AND GIESECKE, AH: *Fluid and electrolyte changes in endocrine disease and their significance in anesthesia.* In BALLINGER, C AND BRECHNER, V (EDS): *Endocrines and Enzymes in Anesthesiology.* Charles C Thomas, Springfield, Illinois, 1973, p 124.

(Urine output continues during surgery if the ECF volume is maintained and bolstered by balanced salt solutions to compensate for that which is translocated incident to the patient's previous trauma or to the manipulations in the surgical procedure. Depletion of ECF resulting from restricted sodium intake or translocations (edema, peritonitis, bowel obstruction, multiple fractures) leads to an increased production of renin, angiotensin, and aldosterone and results in a decreased glomerular filtration.)

94. JENKINS, MT, GIESECKE, AH, AND JOHNSON, ER: *The postoperative patient and his fluid and electrolyte requirements.* Br J Anaesth 47:143, 1975.

(95.) GIESECKE, AH AND JENKINS, MT: *Fluid therapy.* In GIESECKE, AH (ED): *Anesthesia for the Surgery of Trauma.* Clinical Anesthesia Series 11/2, FA Davis, Philadelphia, 1976, p 57.

96. CARRICO, CJ, CANIZARO, PC, AND SHIRES, GT: *Fluid resuscitation following injury: Rationale for the use of balanced salt solutions.* Crit Care Med 4:46, 1976.

(A rational, sensible, and easily applicable approach to the early treatment of hemorrhagic shock, post-injury shock.)

(97.) SHIRES, GT: *Principles and management of hemorrhagic shock.* In SHIRES, GT (ED): *Care of the Trauma Patient,* ed 2. McGraw-Hill, New York, 1979, p 3.

("There is a measurable reduction in the extracellular fluid in response to sustained hemorrhagic shock. It also appears that cellular response to hypovolemic hypotension demonstrates a consistent change in active transport of ions. The evidence obtained directly from living cells indicates that sodium and water enter muscle cells with resultant loss of cellular potassium to the extracellular fluid. The interstitial fluid holds the extruded potassium.")

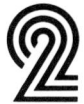

SODIUM BALANCE
R. Dennis Bastron, M.D.

Salt and water balance is the theme of this chapter. Dr. Bastron discusses aspects of this important cation and fluid constituent of the body from the point of view of the clinician. He is eminently qualified to address these issues as he has had a longtime career interest in fluids, electrolytes, and the kidney. The classic hyponatremic incident in anesthesia is the water-overload complication seen occasionally following transurethral resection of the prostate, familiar to all as one of the hallowed Board questions. Hyponatremia is not confined to this dramatic incident by any means. The diagnosis and therapy of the less common syndrome of hypernatremia also is discussed. It is quite apparent that there are a number of etiologic factors which can eventually reduce serum sodium values. Many of these are encountered in the patient who is a candidate for surgery, and consequently, anesthesia. Several formulae for on-the-spot corrections of these deficiencies are explained and placed into clinical context. It is hoped that the background information offered here will assist the clinician to gain better insight and to improve patient care.

Burnell R. Brown, Jr.

Life on earth began about a billion years ago in a sea of moderate salinity which presumably had a composition similar to that of extracellular fluid. Our most primitive ancestors thus had an external milieu similar to our internal milieu. Excretion of wastes was a simple matter for these distant relatives, for they could allow the sea to permeate their tissues, where it would dissolve metabolic waste products, and the solution could be discharged through simple ciliated conduits (Fig. 1).

Approximately 350 million years ago, due perhaps to curiosity or to escape their natural enemies, our ancestors migrated into fresh water streams. This new hypotonic external milieu created a major problem, since they tended to soak up large quantities of water. To survive in fresh water our ancestors developed a relatively impermeable integument and, in addition to their simple excretory conduits, a vascular

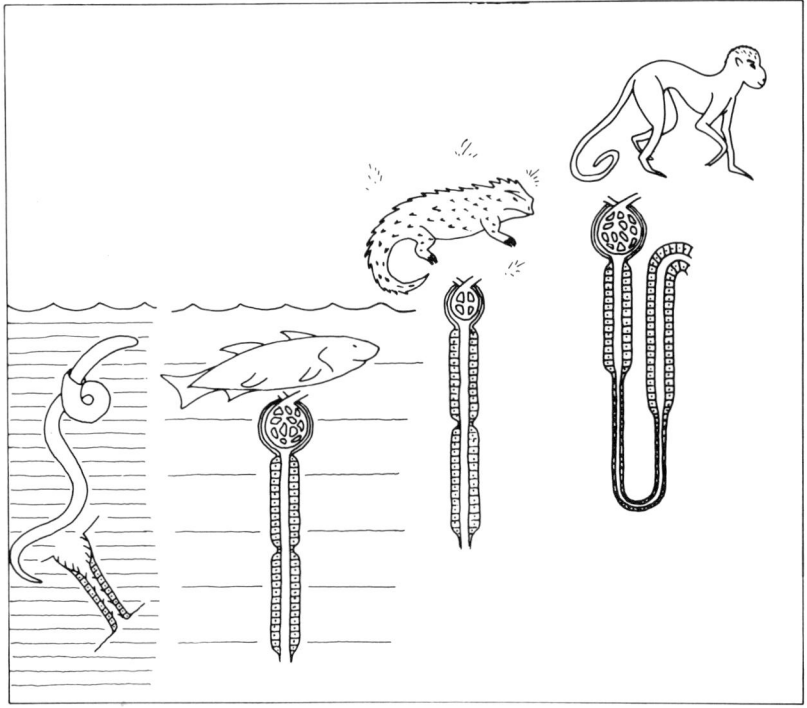

Figure 1. Physiology of the kidney and body fluids. (From Pitts, RF: *Physiology of the Kidney and Body Fluids,* Ed 3. Year Book Medical Publishers, Chicago, 1974, with permission.)

tuft evolved to filter excess water from their bloodstreams. However, filtration created further problems, mainly conservation of valuable solutes present in the filtrate. To conserve these solutes, our fresh water ancestors developed proximal tubules capable of reabsorbing vital compounds and distal tubules capable of diluting urine.

Migration to land 50 million years later produced different problems. Although conservation of sodium and other vital compounds remained important, fluid conservation, rather than fluid elimination, became a major concern. Nitrogen metabolism in reptiles and birds was altered to form uric acid, a relatively insoluble compound, and they developed an efficient tubular secretory mechanism for uric acid. This allowed them to de-emphasize pressure filtration and reduced the number of capillary loops in the glomerular tufts. Mammals, on the other hand, kept their high pressure filtration system and, in addition, developed a counter-current multiplier system which provided the ability to salvage water by concentrating urine. Moreover, sophisticated regulatory control mechanisms were developed to maintain osmolality and extracellular fluid volume.

When renal concentrating and diluting mechanisms are disturbed, the patient will manifest either hyponatremia or hypernatremia. This chapter describes these regulatory mechanisms and outlines an approach to the hyponatremic or hypernatremic patient.

NORMAL TUBULAR FUNCTION

The functional unit of the kidney is the nephron. Figure 2 illustrates the vasculotubular relationships within the kidney, showing that there are at least two classes of nephrons: cortical nephrons and juxtamedullary nephrons. Cortical nephrons outnumber juxtamedullary nephrons approximately 7 to 1 in the human kidney. Cortical nephrons originate from glomeruli in the outer 60 to 75 percent of the cortex and have short loops of Henle which may or may not have a thin segment. The blood supply comes from the afferent arteriole which breaks up to form the glomerular tuft. The capillaries of the glomerular tuft join to form the efferent arteriole, which then divides to form peritubular capillaries. Juxtamedullary nephrons differ from cortical nephrons in several ways. Juxtamedullary glomeruli are larger than cortical glomeruli and have higher single nephron glomerular filtration rates.[1] Juxtamedullary nephrons have long thin loops of Henle which extend deep into the medulla. Efferent arterioles of juxtamedullary nephrons not only form peritubular capillaries but also form vasa recta—long,

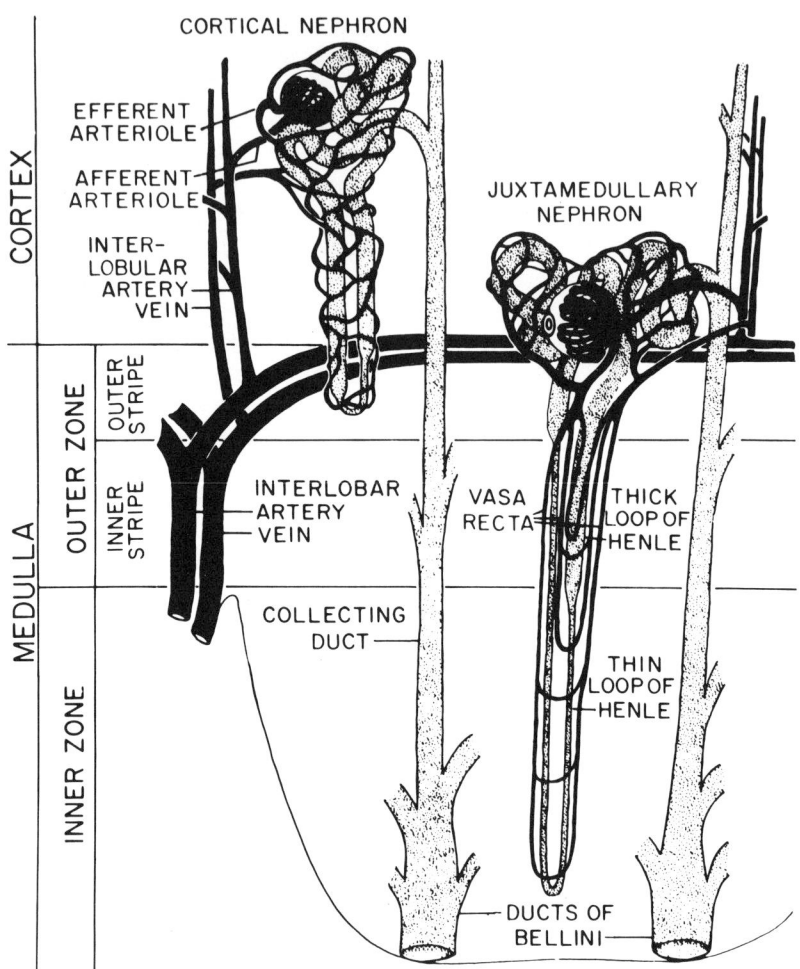

Figure 2. Vasculotubular relationships within the kidney. (From Pitts, RF: *Physiology of the Kidney and Body Fluids,* Ed 3. Year Book Medical Publishers, Chicago, 1974, with permission.)

narrow tubes in a hairpin configuration that accompany the loops of Henle.

The anatomy of the renal circulation contributes to tubular function in several ways. The kidneys are richly perfused, receiving 20 to 25 percent of the cardiac output.[2] There are relatively few branches between the aorta and the afferent arteriole, so that the pressure in the glomerular capillaries is higher than other capillary beds in the body.[3] This large blood flow and high capillary pressure, combined with a very high filtration coefficient of the glomerular capillaries, result in the ultrafiltration of 20 percent of the plasma flowing through a glomeruli to form approximately 180 liters of ultrafiltrate a day. The ratio of the amount of plasma filtered compared with the total plasma flow is known as the filtration fraction, normally 0.20. Since proteins are not filtered, the protein content, and therefore the oncotic pressure, in peritubular capillaries is increased roughly by the same percent as the filtration fraction.

Another way in which the renal circulation contributes to tubular function is related to low hydrostatic pressure in peritubular capillaries. By the time blood enters the peritubular capillaries it has passed through the resistance segments of both the afferent and efferent arterioles, resulting in a hydrostatic pressure lower than in other capillary beds. As will be discussed below, this low hydrostatic pressure in the peritubular capillaries is important in modulating sodium reabsorption in the proximal convoluted tubule.

Finally, the configuration of the vasa recta results in a relatively low medullary blood flow, which is important in maintaining the high medullary interstitial tonicity. In fact, it has been shown that maximum urinary concentrating ability is inversely proportional to medullary blood flow, since an increase in blood flow will tend to "wash out" medullary interstitial solutes and decrease the gradient necessary for urinary concentration.

This 180 liters of filtrate per day must be modified by tubular functions of reabsorption and secretion to form a relatively small volume of urine. Sixty to 70 percent of the filtrate will be reabsorbed in the proximal convoluted tubule (Fig. 3, Mechanism 1). Proximal tubular reabsorption mechanisms are characterized by their ability to transport large volumes, but they are unable to generate large gradients; that is, reabsorption in the proximal convoluted tubule is isosmotic.[4] Current concepts of proximal tubular sodium reabsorption are illustrated in Figure 4. It is now known that there is an active sodium pump located in basolateral membranes of proximal tubular cells. This sodium pump actively transports sodium from within tubular cells into intercellular spaces. This creates a series of concentration, osmotic, pressure, and electrogenic gradients which result in the passive movement of chloride and water from the cells into intercellular spaces; sodium, chloride, and water from tubular fluid into proximal tubular cells; and sodium, chloride, and water from intercellular spaces either

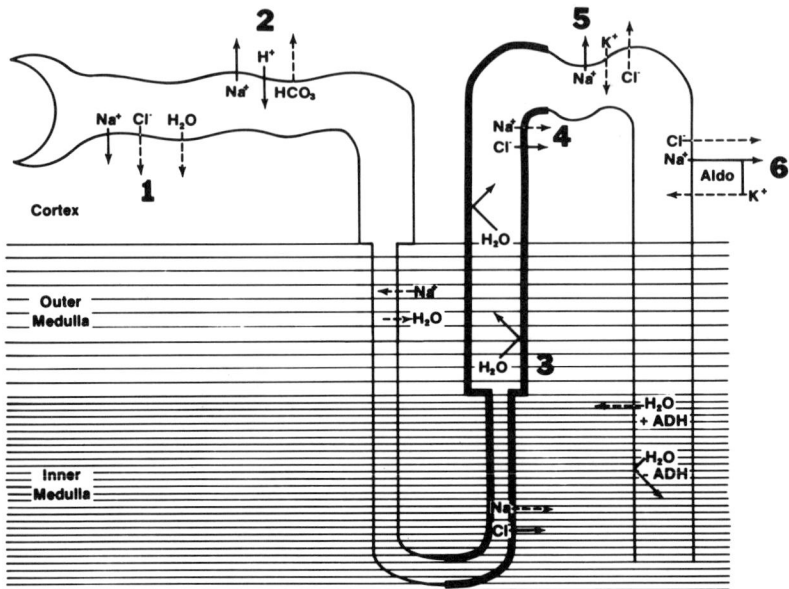

Figure 3. Schematic representation of the major transport processes in the nephron (see text for discussion.) Solid arrows indicate active transport; dashed arrows indicate passive transport. Low permeability is shown as reflected arrows. (From Merin, RG and Bastron RD: *Diuretics.* In Smith, NT, Miller, RD, and Corbascio, AN (eds): *Drug Interactions in Anesthesia.* Lea and Febiger, Philadelphia, 1981, with permission.)

back into the tubule through the "tight junctions" or to be reabsorbed by peritubular capillaries. The amount reabsorbed by peritubular capillaries is influenced by Starling's forces;[5,6] anything that tends to increase colloid osmotic pressure or decrease peritubular capillary pressure will favor reabsorption of salt and water from proximal convoluted tubules, whereas anything that tends to decrease colloid osmotic pressure or increase peritubular capillary hydrostatic pressure will tend to decrease salt reabsorption.

Also in the proximal convoluted tubule are secretory mechanisms for organic acids and bases, and hydrogen ion. The hydrogen ion secretory mechanism is combined with active sodium transport and results in the reabsorption of approximately 80 percent of the bicarbonate from the tubular fluid[7,8] (see Fig. 3, Mechanism 2). By the time tubular fluid reaches the end of the proximal convoluted tubule, therefore, its volume is greatly reduced and its composition altered by reab-

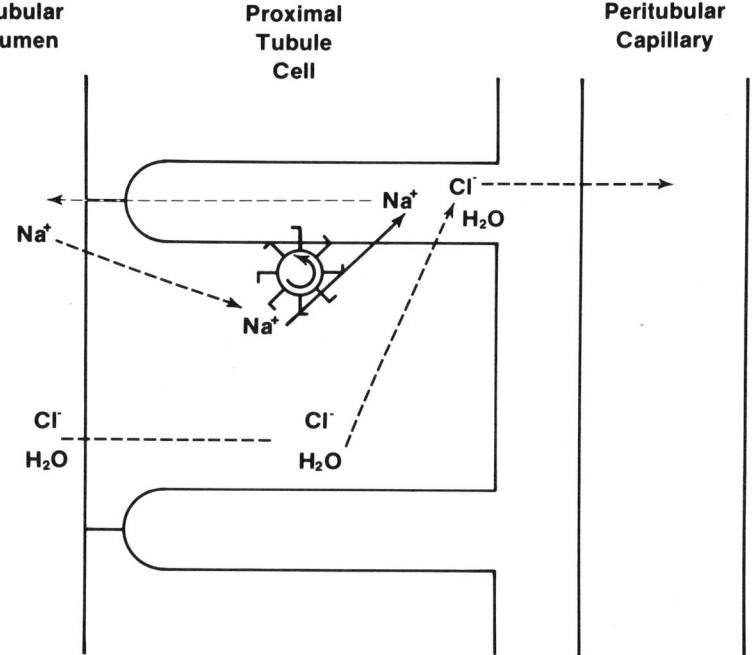

Figure 4. Schematic representation of proximal tubule salt and water reabsorption. (From Merin, RG and Bastron, RD: *Diuretics.* In Smith, NT, Miller, RD, and Corbascio, AN (eds): *Drug Interactions in Anesthesia.* Lea and Febiger, Philadelphia, 1981, with permission.)

sorption of various compounds and secretion of other compounds, yet the osmolality is still about 300 milliosmoles per kilogram of water.

As the fluid enters the descending limb of Henle's loop, it passes down through the medulla, which has increasing interstitial tonicity ranging from approximately 300 milliosmoles per kilogram of water in the outer medulla, reaching a maximum of approximately 1400 milliosmoles per kilogram of water at the tip of the papilla. The epithelium of the descending limb of Henle's loop is permeable to water but relatively impermeable to sodium; water is abstracted from the tubular fluid down an osmotic gradient, resulting in a progressive increase in osmolality of the tubular fluid.[9]

The characteristics of the tubular epithelium change at the bend of the loop—the ascending limb of Henle's loop being relatively impermeable to water.[10] In the thick portion of the ascending limb there is active reabsorption of chloride followed passively by sodium[11] (see Fig. 3, Mechanism 3). Since the tubular epithelium remains relatively impermeable to water, there is a progressive decrease in tubular fluid osmolality and an increase in interstitial osmolality. This segment, the medullary portion of the thick ascending limb of Henle's loop, is known as the concentrating segment of the tubule, since the salt tends to stay in the medullary interstitium (because of the relatively low medullary blood flow), and contributes to the high medullary interstitial tonicity necessary for concentration of urine.

The same process of active chloride and passive sodium reabsorption continues in the cortical portion of the thick limb of Henle's loop (see Fig. 3, Mechanism 4), with a progressive decrease in tubular fluid osmolality until the tubular fluid has an osmolality of approximately 50 milliosmoles per kilogram of water. This segment, the cortical portion of the thick ascending limb of Henle's loop, is therefore known as the diluting segment of the tubule.

In the distal convoluted tubule there again is active transport of sodium. The reabsorptive mechanisms in the distal convoluted tubule are characterized by their ability to transport small volumes of fluid while generating large gradients for a number of compounds, particularly sodium and hydrogen ion (see Fig. 3, Mechanism 5). In late distal convoluted tubule and collecting ducts, there is further reabsorption of sodium, this mechanism (see Fig. 3, Mechanism 6) being under the influence of mineralocorticoids.

In the absence of antidiuretic hormone, the collecting duct is relatively impermeable to water, and a large volume of dilute urine is produced. In the presence of antidiuretic hormone, the collecting duct is freely permeable to water, and water is abstracted down an osmotic gradient produced in the medullary interstitium. The result is a small volume of highly concentrated urine.

FACTORS CONTROLLING SODIUM REABSORPTION

It was originally believed that sodium excretion was determined solely by changes in glomerular filtration rate. Some simple calculations would show that changes in glomerular filtration rate could not be the controlling factor for sodium excretion, however. For example, approximately 15 milliequivalents (mEq) of sodium are filtered each minute and of this 99 percent is reabsorbed, therefore 1 percent is excreted. If the glomerular filtration rate increased by 1 percent, it would double sodium excretion, a condition not compatible with life.

The importance of mineralocorticoids, particularly aldosterone, was then demonstrated. However, the phenomenon known as deoxycorticosterone acetate (DOCA) escape indicated that mineralocortcoids also were not the single controlling factor for sodium reabsorption. This phenomenon can be demonstrated in humans on a constant salt intake by administering DOCA for several days. Initially there will be a marked decrease in salt excretion, with retention of sodium and water, and weight gain. This will last for approximately three to five days, when a new equilibrium will be reached and, in spite of continued DOCA administration, salt excretion will again be equal to salt intake (Fig. 5).

In 1961 de Wardener and associates[12] performed experiments designed to identify the presence of a natriuretic hormone in order to explain the phenomenon of DOCA escape. de Wardener studied dogs receiving chronic DOCA therapy and given large volumes of normal

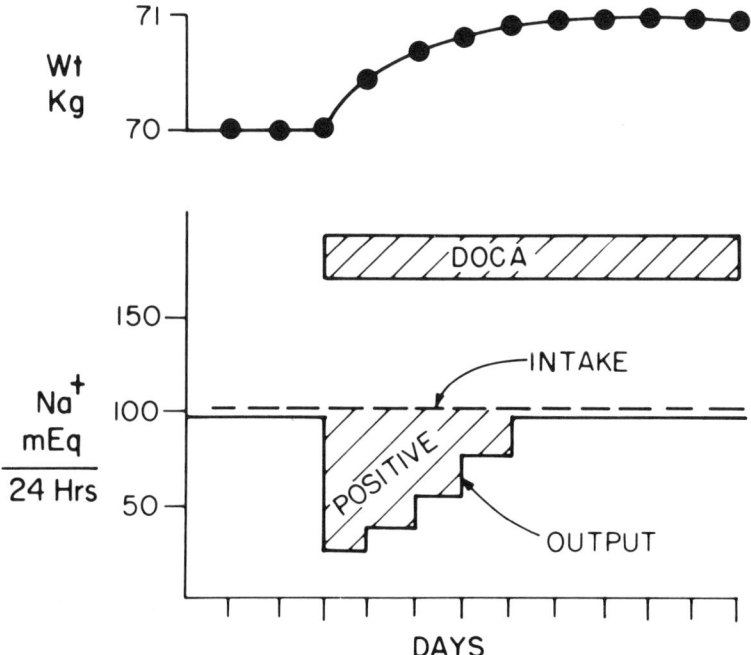

Figure 5. Schematic representation of the "DOCA escape" phenomenon. (From Reineck HJ and Stein JH: *Renal regulation of extracellular fluid volume.* In Brenner, BM and Stein, JH (eds): *Sodium and Water Homeostasis.* Churchill Livingstone, New York, 1978, p 28, with permission.)

saline to produce volume expansion. Simultaneously, renal arterial pressure was decreased by constricting the aorta to produce a slight decrease in glomerular filtration rate. Despite the decreased glomerular filtration rate and constant mineralocorticoid influence, a natriuresis was produced. While these results were interpreted as demonstrating the presence of "third factor" or natriuretic hormone, the experiments stimulated other investigators to look at different mechanisms to explain the results. It has now been demonstrated that changes in Starling's forces probably account for de Wardener's findings (see below). Kaloyanides and Azer,[13] however, have demonstrated the presence of natriuretic hormone in dogs. An as yet unidentified natriuretic hormone appears to be present in humans, particularly in patients with chronic renal failure.[14] It is doubtful, however, that natriuretic hormone plays a role in sodium homeostasis in health.

Starling's forces in peritubular capillaries have been demonstrated to play a major role in sodium reabsorption in proximal convoluted tubules. In a variety of experiments designed to explain de Wardener's results, it has been shown that sodium reabsorption is favored by increased peritubular capillary oncotic pressure and a low hydrostatic pressure.[5,6] Oncotic pressure may increase because of increases in serum albumin. An increase in filtration fraction, commonly seen during anesthesia or hypotension, will also increase oncotic pressure in peritubular capillaries. Peritubular capillary hydrostatic pressure may decrease with systemic hypotension. Systemic hypertension and dilution of body fluids with a fall in serum albumin will result in changes in Starling's forces, which tend to decrease salt reabsorption in proximal convoluted tubule.

Medullary blood flow as a determinate of sodium reabsorption was first postulated by Earley and Friedler in 1964.[15] The rationale is as follows: Increased medullary blood flow will cause a fall in interstitial hypertonicity of the medulla, which will result in less water abstraction from the descending limb of Henle's loop. This will necessarily cause increased delivery of salt and water to distal segments of the tubule. If there is a time-gradient limited salt pump it would therefore increase salt excretion. While this hypothesis is attractive, it has not been adequately tested in an experimental model.

Barger and his colleagues,[16,17] in a series of experiments, demonstrated that a number of experimental conditions associated with salt retention were also associated with redistribution of blood flow from outer cortex to inner cortex and medulla, as demonstrated by inert gas washout curves and by microfil injections of the renal vessels. They postulated that the cortical nephrons were relative salt losers, and the juxtamedullary nephrons, with their long loops of Henle, were relative salt retainers. Stein and coworkers,[18] and Bastron and associates,[19] however, using different experimental models and using microspheres to estimate the distribution of blood flow within the kidney, have demonstrated increased inner cortical blood flow associated with natriuresis. Thus, it is not clear whether the characterization of juxtamedullary nephrons as salt retainers is valid.

Sympathetic nerve activity is known to modulate sodium excretion. Denervation ordinarily results in increased sodium excretion, while increased sympathetic activity is normally associated with decreased sodium excretion. It is possible that sympathetic nerve activity influences sodium excretion by altering the hemodynamic mechanisms discussed above. However, recent studies have demonstrated[20] alterations in sodium excretion with low levels of renal nerve stimulation which are insufficient to influence renal blood flow, glomerular filtration rate, perfusion pressure, or intrarenal distribution of blood flow. These findings, in conjunction with the recent demonstration of sympathetic nerve endings on proximal tubule cells,[21] suggest that sympathetic nerve activity may indeed play a role in the modulation of sodium balance independent of hemodynamically induced changes.

CONCENTRATION AND DILUTION OF URINE

The ability to concentrate and dilute urine obviously is important to mammals. An average-sized man can excrete a 1-liter water load in 2 to 3 hours by diluting his urine to approximately 50 milliosmoles per kilogram of water. Compulsive water drinkers can excrete 20 to 30 liters of free water a day. Water deprivation, on the other hand, is accommodated for by concentrating urine to a maximum of approximately 1200 to 1400 milliosmoles per kilogram of water, with a normal daily solute load being excreted in 400 milliliters of highly concentrated urine. Factors necessary for the dilution of urine include adequate fluid delivery to the ascending limb of Henle's loop, normal ascending limb function (which results in a low tubular fluid osmolality and high medullary interstitial osmolality), and normal collecting duct function (and the absence of antidiuretic hormone). For urinary concentration, in addition to these factors, there must be a relatively low medullary blood flow and the presence of antidiuretic hormone (ADH) or drugs with a similar effect.

Inadequate delivery of fluid to Henle's loop occurs in hypotension and shock because of decreased glomerular filtration and enhanced proximal tubular reabsorption of salt and water. Hypotension produces decreased renal blood flow and glomerular filtration rate through a variety of neural and humoral mechanisms. The decrease in glomerular filtration ordinarily is less than the decrease in renal blood flow, therefore resulting in an increased filtration fraction. Increased filtration fraction in turn results in increased oncotic pressure in peritubular capillaries. The decreased systemic blood pressure and increased resistance in the afferent arterioles are reflected in decreased hydrostatic pressure in peritubular capillaries. These alterations in Starling's forces in peritubular capillaries enhance proximal tubular reabsorption.

Acute renal failure (acute tubular necrosis) also results in decreased glomerular filtration, and may also impair fluid delivery to Henle's loop secondary to backleak of fluid out of damaged tubules[22] or to tubular obstruction by casts.[23]

Ascending limb (concentrating and diluting segments) function is most often impaired by "loop" diuretics, thiazides, and osmotic diuresis from glucose, mannitol or urea. "Abnormal" collecting duct function in diluting defects (causing hyponatremia) is commonly related to unusual ADH release, production of substances with activity similar to ADH (e.g., lung tumors), or administration of drugs with properties similar to ADH. The action of ADH on collecting ducts to cause urinary concentration is inhibited by lithium and inorganic fluoride (methoxyflurane toxicity).

Both water diuresis and mannitol appear to increase medullary blood flow, and therefore decrease maximal concentrating ability.

ADH is produced in magnocellular neurons in the supraoptic and paraventricular nuclei and released from the neural lobe of the pituitary. In addition to decreasing water and urea permeability of the collecting duct, ADH is a vasoconstrictor, decreases renal renin release, and may influence memory and corticotropin release.[24] Perhaps the primary mechanism for stimulating the release of ADH is osmolality (i.e., so-called osmoreceptors), and a direct relationship between plasma osmolality and ADH release has been demonstrated in a variety of animals under many different conditions.[24]

Baroreceptors in the aortic arch and carotid sinus also influence ADH release. Left atrial baroreceptors (Gauer-Henry reflexes) influence extracellular fluid volume in some species, but appear to be relatively unimportant in primates.[25] Baroreceptors in the juxtaglomerular apparatuses influence ADH release via the renin-angiotensin system.

Should osmoreceptors and baroreceptors act in opposite directions (e.g., decreased osmolality tending to decrease ADH release and hypotension tending to increase ADH release), the baroreceptor response appears to override the osmoreceptor effect.[24] (This may merely reflect a change in the intercept, without a change in the slope of the response curve of ADH release to osmotic stimulation.) Pain and stress can produce ADH release (possibly via endorphins) in the face of hypo-osmolality as can nausea and vomiting. Hypothermia decreases, and hyperthermia increases, ADH release. Hypothyroidism and adrenal insufficiency may be associated with increased ADH levels.

Thus, while osmotic stimuli are the most sensitive determinants of ADH release, they can be overridden by nonosmotic influences of greater magnitude.

CLINICAL APPROACH TO THE HYPONATREMIC OR HYPERNATREMIC PATIENT

Aberrations in urinary concentrating or diluting mechanisms ordinarily result in hyponatremia or hypernatremia. I have found the approach of Berl and Schrier[26] to the hyponatremic patient to be simple and useful. First, it is incumbent upon the physician to be certain that the blood sample was not improperly drawn, for example from a site proximal to a hypotonic saline or dextrose infusion. Pseudohyponatremia must also be ruled out. Pseudohyponatremia can occur with severe hyperlipidemia (associated with diabetic ketoacidosis or hypothyroidism) or severe hyperproteinemia (e.g., with multiple myeloma or Waldenstrom's macroglobulinemia). A pathologically high concentration of fats or proteins occupies a larger portion of plasma, thereby decreasing the amount of water contained in the plasma. In pseudohyponatremia, the concentration of sodium in total plasma is low, but the concentration of sodium in plasma water is normal.

Serum osmolality can be calculated by using the formula:

$$Osm = 2Na(mEq/liter) + \frac{glucose\ (mg/dl)}{18} + \frac{urea\ nitrogen\ (mg/dl)}{2.8}$$

Serum osmolality estimated by this formula should differ by no more than 10 milliosmoles per kilogram of water from directly measured serum osmolality. Elevations in serum glucose or urea should be reflected in a decreased serum sodium if osmolality is to remain normal, and a low serum sodium under those circumstances should not be considered as primary hyponatremia. For example, one would expect serum sodium to decrease approximately 1.6 mEq per liter for each 100 mg per dl increase in serum glucose[27] and similarly serum sodium should decrease approximately 1.2 mEq per liter for each 10 mg per dl increase in blood urea nitrogen.[28] Moreover, serum sodium may be decreased in the presence of large concentrations of other nonreabsorbable solutes such as mannitol.

When satisfied that the patient is indeed hyponatremic, an effort should be made to determine whether the patient's extracellular fluid volume is expanded, contracted, or normal, and urinary sodium concentration (Una) should be measured (see Table 1 later in this section). The volume contracted patient will show signs of postural hypotension, tachycardia, poor skin turgor, and low central venous pressure or pulmonary capillary wedge pressure. This patient also has a deficit of both sodium and water with a greater deficit of sodium. Since the normal renal response to volume contraction is sodium retention, the finding of urinary sodium concentration of less than 20 mEq per liter points to extrarenal losses as a route for sodium and water loss. This would most commonly be either through the gastrointestinal tract (vomiting or diarrhea, nasogastric suctioning, and so forth), or from so-called "third space" losses such as seen in surgical and nonsurgical trauma, burns, pancreatitis, and peritonitis. Urinary sodium concentrations greater than 20 mEq per liter point to renal losses of the salt and water. In surgical patients the most common cause of renal losses with volume contraction are excessive use of "loop" diuretic agents, or osmotic diuresis from hyperglycemia, uremia, or mannitol. Less common causes include mineralocorticoid deficiencies, salt-losing nephropathies, renal tubular acidosis with bicarbonaturia, and severe metabolic alkalosis with bicarbonaturia.

Expanded extracellular fluid volume is characterized by edema. Edematous, hyponatremic patients have an increase in total body sodium and total body water with a proportionately greater increase in the total water. Edematous, hyponatremic patients with urinary sodium concentrations greater than 20 mEq per liter ordinarily are suffering from either acute or chronic renal failure. Urinary sodium concentrations of less than 20 mEq per liter in edematous, hyponatremic patients ordinarily are associated with congestive heart failure, cirrhosis or, less frequently in surgical patients, the nephrotic syndrome (Table 1).

Table 1. Causes of hyponatremia

Serum sodium < 135 mEq/liter			
Volume contracted (salt loss in excess of water loss)		*"Euvolemic"*	*Edematous* (water retention in excess of salt retention)
Una < 20 mEq/liter (extrarenal losses)	Una > 20 mEq/liter (renal losses)		Una < 20 mEq/liter / Una > 20 mEq/liter
Gastrointestinal	Diuretic excess	Stress	Cardiac failure / Renal failure
vomiting	Osmotic diuresis	physical	Cirrhosis / acute
diarrhea	glucose	emotional	Nephrotic syndrome / chronic
suction	urea	Transurethral resection	
fistula drainage	mannitol	Antidiuretic drugs*	
"Third space" losses	radiographic contrast material	SIADH†	
burns		Diuretics with hypokalemia	
peritonitis	Mineralocorticoid deficiency	Glucocorticoid deficiency	
trauma		Hypothyroidism	
pancreatitis	Salt-losing nephritis		
bowel obstruction	Bicarbonaturia with tubular acidosis		
	metabolic alkalosis		

*See Table 2.
†Syndrome of inappropriate antidiuretic hormone secretion.
(Modified from Berl, T and Schrier, RW: *Water metabolism and the hypo-osmolar syndromes*. In Brenner, BM and Stein, JH (eds): *Sodium and Water Homeostasis*. Churchill Livingstone, New York, 1978, p 1.)

Patients who are hyponatremic, but are neither volume contracted nor edematous, usually will have one of the conditions listed in Table 1. Of the causes listed in the differential diagnosis of hyponatremia in the clinically euvolemic patient, the most common causes in surgical patients are physical or emotional stress; transurethral resection; antidiuretic drugs (Table 2), particularly morphine, oxytocin and vasopressin derivatives used in obstetrics; and finally, the syndrome of inappropriate ADH secretion. It should be noted that the syndrome of inappropriate ADH secretion is a diagnosis made by exclusion. The criteria for diagnosis of the syndrome of inappropriate ADH secretion are listed in Table 3.

The signs and symptoms of hyponatremia usually begin with anorexia, confusion, headaches, and muscle cramps, progressing to nausea, vomiting, and personality changes, and finally to convulsions, coma, and death. The signs and symptoms are not well correlated

Table 2. Drugs with antidiuretic properties

Nicotine	Vincristine
Chlorpropamide	Carbamazepine
Tolbutamide	Acetaminophen
Clofibrate	Indomethacin
Cyclophosphamide	Isoproterenol
Morphine	Oxytocin
Barbiturates	Vasopressin

(Modified from Berl, T and Schrier, RW: *Water metabolism and the hypo-osmolar syndromes.* In Brenner, BM and Stein, JH (eds): *Sodium and Water Homeostasis.* Churchill Livingstone, New York, 1978, p 1.)

Table 3. Criteria for the diagnosis of SIADH

1. Hyponatremia with hypo-osmolality.
2. Inappropriately concentrated urine containing large quantities of sodium.
3. Absence of azotemia, edema, or signs of decreased extracellular fluid volume.
4. Normal endocrine function.
5. Correction of hyponatremia with rigid restriction of water intake.

(Adapted from Deutsch, S, Goldberg, M, and Dripps RD: *Postoperative hyponatremia with inappropriate release of antidiuretic hormone.* Anesthesiology 27:250, 1966) with the degree of hyponatremia, but appear to be more common with more rapidly developing hyponatremia rather than chronic hyponatremia. A patient with suddenly occurring hyponatremia may become symptomatic at sodium levels of 128 to 130 mEq per liter, whereas with slowly developing hyponatremia, patients may be relatively asymptomatic with serum sodium levels of less than 120 mEq per liter.

Acute hyponatremia is associated with a mortality rate exceeding 50 percent. Chronic symptomatic hyponatremia has a lower, but still significant, mortality rate—approaching 10 percent—whereas chronic, asymptomatic hyponatremia is associated with a very low mortality rate.[29] It has recently been shown that relatively low levels of hyponatremia for even a short period of time can be associated with death or permanent neurologic sequelae.[30] Thus, hyponatremia is a serious condition which needs aggressive and rational therapy.

TREATMENT OF HYPONATREMIA

It is generally agreed that patients with severe neurologic symptoms, that is, convulsions or coma secondary to hyponatremia, should be vigorously treated with the administration of hypertonic saline. The amount of sodium required can be calculated by subtracting the patient's measured serum sodium from 140 mEq per liter and multiplying that figure times the patient's weight in kilograms times 0.6 (to calculate total body water). It is known that sodium is distributed primarily in the extracellular fluid. However, the osmolality must be corrected in total body water; therefore, the calculation corrects for total body water rather than extracellular fluid water. The calculated total requirement of milliequivalents of sodium should then be given in the form of 3 or 5 percent sodium chloride with half the calculated requirement given the first 8 hours with frequent reassessment. Treatment should be continued until neurologic symptoms resolve or until a serum sodium of 130 mEq per liter is achieved. In most hyponatremic patients, an infusion at a rate of 1 mEq of sodium per kilogram body weight per hour will raise serum sodium 2 to 3 mEq per liter per hour.[29] Another simple rule of thumb is that the patient's weight in kg $\times$ 6 = the number of ml of 5 percent sodium chloride required to increase serum sodium by 10 mEq per liter[31] (see reference for the derivation). The main hazards of rapid correction of hyponatremia with hypertonic saline are fluid overload (pulmonary edema), and convulsions if serum sodium (osmolality) increases too rapidly.

Case report: A 68-year-old, 52 kg woman was admitted to the SICU after having a grand mal seizure and respiratory arrest. She was 5 days postmitral valve replacement. She had done well for 48 hours and was transferred to an intermediate care area. Over the next 3 days she became progressively lethargic until the seizure. Review of her chart revealed she had been receiving only 2000 ml of D5W daily since transfer. She had been unable to resume oral intake. Her serum sodium was 109 mEq per liter and her urinary sodium was 70 mEq per liter. The patient was comatose and flaccid on admission to the SICU. Her sodium deficit was calculated to be 967 mEq (140−109 × 52 × 0.6). She was given 60 mEq of sodium per hour (967 × 0.5 ÷ 8) in addition to calculated maintenance fluids. Within 5 hours she regained consciousness and adequate spontaneous ventilation. At that time her serum sodium was 121 mEq per liter. With fluid restriction and continued replacement of urinary and gastric salt losses, her electrolytes and physical status returned to normal 48 hours after admission.

Patients who do not have severe neurologic symptoms should be treated more conservatively—by fluid restriction. Ordinarily, limiting the patient's fluid intake to less than a liter per day will result in correction of the hyponatremia over a period of several days. Should there be more urgency in correcting hyponatremia, another method can be used which was described by Hantmen and colleagues.[32] These investigators use furosemide to induce a negative water balance, the urinary electrolytes being replaced with intravenous sodium and potassium. An example of this method is shown in Figure 6.

The amount of total negative water balance necessary to correct the hyponatremia can be calculated as follows. The patient's total body water is calculated by multiplying the weight in kilograms times 0.6. That figure is then multiplied by the ratio of the deviation of the patient's serum sodium from normal serum sodium to calculate the amount of excess body water needed to excrete to have a normal serum sodium.

Example: 70 kg patient, serum Na = 126 mEq per liter.
a) Total body water = 42 liters (70 × 0.6)
b) Ratio of deviation of sodium =
$$\frac{\text{normal Na} - \text{serum Na}}{\text{normal Na}} = \frac{140 - 126}{140} = 0.10$$
c) Excess fluid = 42 liters × 0.10 = 4.2 liters.

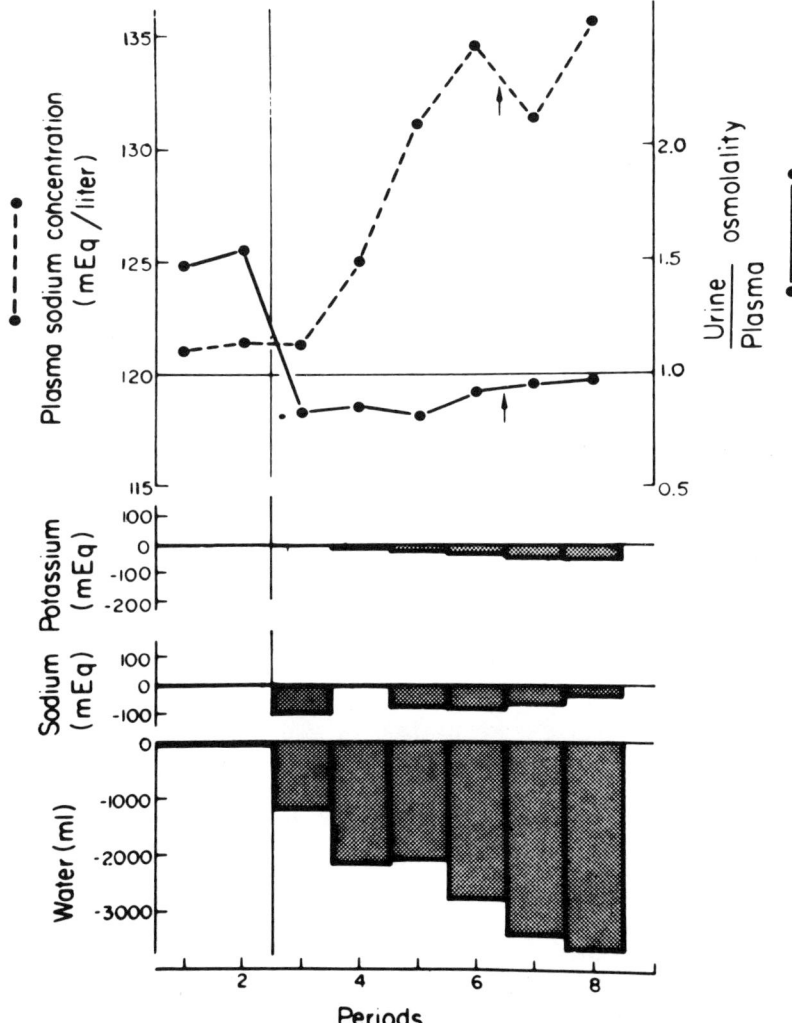

Figure 6. Graphs for method of rapidly correcting symptomatic hyponatremia by inducing a negative water balance with a loop diuretic as urinary electrolyte losses are replaced. Furosemide administered at 2½ periods (vertical line) and at 6½ periods (arrow). Negative water balance *(bottom)* and not a positive sodium or potassium balance *(middle)* accounted for the rise in plasma sodium concentration *(top)*. (From Hantman, D, et al: *Rapid correction of hyponatremia in the syndrome of inappropriate secretion of antidiuretic hormone: An alternative treatment to hypertonic saline.* Adv Intern Med 78:870, 1973, with permission.)

It is paramount, however, while correcting the patient's serum sodium that the underlying disorder be corrected as well. While certain drugs such as lithium and demococycline have been used to treat water retaining disorders, their safety has not been shown to be equal to the more conservative therapy of water deprivation.

HYPERNATREMIA

Hypernatremia occurs when there is loss of water in excess of sodium loss, or under certain circumstances when there is excessive salt intake. In infants, acute hypernatremia may occur because of accidental ingestion of salt formula in place of sugar formula. Chronic hypernatremia in children may occur from any of the causes listed in Table 4, the most common being gastroenteritis or infection. Acute hypernatremia may occur in adults secondary to misadventures during hypertonic saline abortion, overuse of saline as an emetic, hemodialysis malfunction, heat stroke, salt water near-drowning, and the use of large doses of sodium bicarbonate in the treatment of cardiac arrest or metabolic acidosis. Chronic hypernatremia in adults may occur from any of the causes listed in Table 5.

The symptoms of hypernatremia are primarily related to the nervous system, including irritability, which can progress to convulsions and death. In children the mortality rate of acute hypernatremia is in

Table 4. Causes of chronic hypernatremia in children

Loss of water in excess of sodium
Gastroenteritis.
Infection causing anorexia, fever, and tachypnea.
Diabetic ketoacidosis.
Diabetes insipidus with limited access to water.
Primary CNS disease limiting water intake.
Osmotic agents (mannitol, radiographic contrast agents).

Excessive salt intake
Improper feeding formulas.

(From Covey, CM and Arieff, AI: *Disorders of sodium and water metabolism and their effects on the central nervous system.* In Brenner, BM and Stein, JH (eds): *Sodium and Water Homeostasis.* Churchill Livingstone, New York, 1978, with permission.)

Table 5. Causes of chronic hypernatremia in adults

Infirmity with inability to replace water losses.
Impaired thirst mechanism.
Renal water loss with inadequate replacement.
  Solute-induced
    Diuretic phase of ATN, postobstruction, or renal transplantation.
    High solute feedings.
    Diabetes mellitus.
    Mannitol or urea infusion.
    Diabetes insipidus with failure of thirst response.
    Chronic renal failure.
Large insensible losses, inadequately replaced
  Dehydration in warm climates.
  Fever and hyperventilation.
Other
  Excessive water removal with dialysis.
  Steroid excess.

(From Covey, CM and Arieff, AI: *Disorders of sodium and water metabolism and their effects on the central nervous system.* In Brenner, BM and Stein, JH (eds): *Sodium and Water Homeostasis.* Churchill Livingstone, New York, 1978, p 215, with permission.)

excess of 40 percent, and in chronic hypernatremia it approaches 10 percent.[29] In adults acute hypernatremia (serum sodium greater than 160 mEq per liter) is associated with a 70 percent mortality rate whereas chronic hypernatremia is associated with a 60 percent mortality rate.[29] The water deficit in a hypernatremic patient can be calculated by multiplying the total body water times the ratio of the deviation of serum sodium from normal.

Example: 70 kg patient, serum Na = 154 mEq per liter.
a) Total body water = 70 × 0.6 − 42 liters
b) Percent deviation of sodium =
$$\frac{\text{serum Na} - \text{normal}}{\text{normal sodium}} = \frac{154 - 140}{140} = 0.10$$
c) Water deficit = 42 liters × 0.10 = 4.2 liters.

The treatment of hypernatremia includes the following steps: (1) If the patient is in shock, resuscitate with crystalloids or colloids to stabilize the cardiovascular system. (2) Treat acidosis with sodium bicarbonate, only if the pH is less than 7.20. (3) Estimate the fluid deficit and replace with hypotonic fluid. This replacement should take place over 48 hours with a goal of decreasing serum osmolality by no more than 2 milliosmoles per hour. Note that this deficit should be replaced in addition to maintenance fluids and continuing fluid losses. Plasma sodium or osmolality should be measured approximately every two hours. (4) Always remember to treat the underlying disease!

The best fluid for correcting hypernatremia in adults is not known. In children, however, a solution consisting of one-fifth normal saline and 2½ percent glucose has been shown to correct hypernatremia with a minimal amount of posttreatment edema; 5 percent glucose appears to cause a high incidence of pitting edema; and one-half normal saline is less effective in correcting the hypernatremia.

Case report: A 22-year-old male was admitted because of lassitude, weakness, headache, and confusion which developed while playing tennis during midday. Ambient temperature was 107°F Patient's oral temperature was 40.5°C, BP 95/55 torr, P 124 beats/min, Hct 50% and serum sodium 155 mEq per liter. The patient normally weighed 82 kg. (He weighed 78 kg on admission.) His calculated water deficit was 5.4 liters (82 kg $\times$ 0.60 = 49.2 liters body water; 155 − 140 $\div$ 140 = 0.11; 49.2 $\times$ 0.11 = 5.4 liters deficit). His urine output and calculated insensible losses were replaced with one-half normal saline in 5 percent glucose. In addition he received one-fifth normal saline in 2½ percent glucose at a rate of 125 ml/hr. After 18 hours his symptoms resolved (serum sodium 148 mEq per liter) and his intravenous therapy was discontinued. His electrolytes were normal after another 18 hours on oral intake.

REFERENCES

1. Jamison, RL: *Evidence for functional intrarenal heterogeneity obtained by micropuncture technique.* Yale J Biol Med 45:254, 1972.
2. Hollenberg, NK: *The renal circulation.* In Zelis R: *The Peripheral Circulations.* Grune and Stratton, New York, 1975, p 131.
3. Brenner, BM, Troy, JL, and Daugharty, TM: *The dynamics of glomerular ultra-filtration in the rat.* J Clin Invest 50:1776, 1971.
4. Reineck, HJ and Stein, JH: *Renal regulation of extracellular fluid volume.* In Brenner, BM and Stein, JH: *Sodium and Water Homeostasis.* Churchill Livingstone, New York, 1978, p 240.

5. BRENNER, BM, TROY, JL, AND DAUGHARTY, TM: *On the mechanism of inhibition of fluid reabsorption by the renal proximal tubule of the volume expanded rat.* J Clin Invest 50:1596, 1971.
6. BRENNER, BM, TROY, JL, AND DAUGHARTY, TM: *Quantitative importance of changes in postglomerular colloid osmotic pressure in mediating glomerular tubular balance in the rat.* J Clin Invest 52:190, 1973.
7. GOTTSCHALK, CW, LASSITER, WE, AND MYLLE, M: *Localization of urine acidification in the mammalian kidney.* Am J Physiol 198:581, 1960.
8. RECTOR, FC, JR, CARTER, NW, AND SELDIN, DW: *The mechanism of bicarbonate reabsorption in the proximal and distal tubules of the kidney.* J Clin Invest 44:278, 1965.
9. KOKKO, JP: *Sodium chloride and water transport in the descending limb of Henle.* J Clin Invest 49:1838, 1979.
10. IMAI, M AND KOKKO, JP: *Sodium chloride, urea and water transport in the thin ascending limb of Henle. Generation of osmotic gradients by passive diffusion of solutes.* J Clin Invest 53:393, 1974.
11. BURG, MB, ET AL: *Furosemide effect on isolated perfused tubules.* Am J Physiol 225:119, 1973.
12. DE WARDENER, HE, ET AL: *Studies on the efferent mechanism of the sodium diuresis which follows the administration of intravenous saline in the dog.* Clinical Science 21:249, 1961.
13. KALOYANIDES, GJ AND AZER, M: *Evidence for a humoral mechanism in volume expansion natriuresis.* J Clin Invest 50:1603, 1971.
14. BRICKER, NS, ET AL: *On the biology of sodium excretion: The search for a natriuretic hormone.* Yale J Biol Med 48:293, 1975.
15. EARLEY, LE AND FRIEDLER, RM: *Observations on the mechanism of decreased tubular reabsorption of sodium and water during saline loading.* J Clin Invest 43:1928, 1964.
16. BARGER, AC: *Renal hemodynamic factors in congestive heart failure.* Ann NY Acad Sci 139:276, 1966.
17. BARGER, AC AND HERD, JA: *The renal circulation.* N Engl J Med 284:482, 1971.
18. STEIN, JH, ET AL: *Effect of renal vasodilation on the distribution of cortical blood flow in the kidney of the dog.* J Clin Invest 50:1429, 1971.
19. BASTRON, RD, PYNE, JL, AND INAGAKI, M: *Halothane-induced renal vasodilation.* Anesthesiology 50:126, 1979.
20. SLICK, GL, ET AL: *Renal neuroadrenergic transmission.* Am J Physiol 229:60, 1975.
21. MULLER, J AND BARAJAS, L: *Electron microscopic and histochemical evidence for a tubular innervation in the renal cortex of the monkey.* J Ultrastruct Res 41:533, 1972.

22. BANK, N, MUTZ, FG, AND AYNEDJIAN, HS: *The role of "leakage" of tubular fluid in anuria due to mercury poisoning.* J Clin Invest 46:695, 1967.
23. ARENDSHORST, WJ, FINN, WF, AND GOTTSCHALK, CW: *Pathogenesis of acute renal failure following temporary renal ischemia in the rat.* Circ Res 37:558, 1975.
24. WEITZMAN, RE: *Factors regulating the secretion and metabolism of arginine vasopressin (antidiuretic hormone).* In BRENNER, BM AND STEIN, JH (EDS): *Hormonal Function and the Kidney.* Churchill Livingstone, New York, 1979, p 146.
25. GILMORE, JP AND ZUCKER, IH: *Failure of left atrial distention to alter renal function in the nonhuman primate.* Circ Res 42:267, 1978.
26. BERL, T AND SCHRIER, RW: *Water metabolism and the hypo-osmolar syndromes.* In BRENNER, BM AND STEIN, JH (EDS): *Sodium and Water Homeostasis.* Churchill Livingstone, New York, 1978, p 1.
27. KATZ, MA: *Hyperglycemia-induced hyponatremia—calculation of expected serum sodium depression.* N Engl J Med 289:843, 1973.
28. GOLDBERGER, E: *A Primer of Water, Electrolyte and Acid-Base Syndromes,* ed 5. Lea and Febiger, Philadelphia, 1975, p 590.
29. COVEY, CM AND ARIEFF, AI: *Disorders of sodium and water metabolism and their effects on the central nervous system.* In BRENNER, BM AND STEIN, JH (EDS): *Sodium and Water Homeostasis.* Churchill Livingstone, New York, 1978, p 212.
30. ARIEFF, AI AND WITTE, JM: *Death or permanent neurological disability despite correction of protracted hyponatremia* (abstr). Am Soc Nephrol 185A, 1979.
31. GOLDBERGER, E: *A Primer of Water, Electrolyte and Acid-Base Syndromes,* ed 5. Lea and Febiger, Philadelphia, 1975, p 584.
32. HANTMAN, D, ET AL: *Rapid correction of hyponatremia in the syndrome of inappropriate secretion of antidiuretic hormone: An alternative to hypertonic saline.* Adv Intern Med 78:870, 1973.

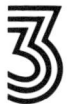

BALANCED SALT SOLUTIONS IN MASSIVE TRAUMA

C. James Carrico, M.D., and
Ronald V. Maier, M.D.

Drs. Maier and Carrico are surgeons with particular interests in trauma and fluid balance. Dr. Carrico was a resident under Dr. G. Tom Shires, an intrepid researcher in extracellular fluid spaces and an advocate for restoration of this space during surgery. In this chapter current concepts of interstitial extracellular water shifts are reviewed.

There are three sources of interstitial fluid loss associated with shock, hemorrhage, and trauma. In the first of these, the reservoir of interstitial extracellular fluid is called upon to replace plasma volume diminished by hemorrhage. Until Shires' studies, it was not appreciated that as hemorrhage occurs, the body rapidly swings its volume of interstitial fluid into the vascular tree. This interstitial blood must eventually be replaced. A second site of loss is tissue edema: removing interstitial fluid from its functional compartment. Tissue edema is due to both the initial trauma and to the trauma produced by surgery. Long intraperitoneal procedures cause significant fluid translocations into gut and peritoneal wall edema. The third site of loss is into tissue cells (primarily skeletal muscle), due to diminished activity of the membrane sodium pump with decreased perfusion. This leads to a "running down" of the cellular gradient so that an electric membrane potential change occurs as sodium enters the cell and potassium leaves. The hydration number of a sodium ion is three. That is, three water molecules enter the cell with every sodium ion.

These sources of loss dictate replacement with a balanced salt solution mimicking interstitial extracellular fluid. Ringer's lactate is commonly used. It must be emphasized that use of Ringer's lactate is not meant to replace blood. It is a replacement of extracellular fluid.

Burnell R. Brown, Jr.

The need for fluid resuscitation in the massively traumatized patient occurs because of depletion in the intravascular and extravascular, extracellular volumes secondary to losses induced by the injuries. The amount of these losses and the necessity for appropriate replacement increase in proportion to the extent of the trauma incurred. Inability to stop loss of volume or replace loss rapidly, or both, leads to the pathophysiologic state commonly referred to as hypovolemic shock. The ability to express physiologically what shock means to the patient has developed slowly over the past 100 years. Until the late 1800s, many defined shock as a normal physiologic state following injury and felt that it should not be altered. Gross, in 1872, was one of the first to challenge this concept, and defined shock as "the manifestation of the rude unhinging of the machinery of life."[1] Further clarification of the physiology underlying the shock state was supplied by Blalock in 1940: "shock is a peripheral circulatory failure resulting from a discrepancy in the size of the vascular bed and the volume of the intravascular fluid."[2] Current concepts define shock as a manifestation of inadequate tissue perfusion with low flow states in vital organs, which is the final common denominator in all forms of shock.[3]

Shock or hypoperfusion at the tissue level may be induced by multiple mechanisms. Simply, these may be defined as: (1) *Cardiogenic shock:* failure of the heart as a pump brought about by primary myocardial dysfunction—may be induced by myocardial infarction, cardiac arrhythmias, or myocardial depression secondary to multiple etiologies or other causes which restrict the ability of the myocardium to pump (i.e., tension pneumothorax, vena cava obstruction, or cardiac tamponade); (2) *Hypovolemic shock:* reduction in the fluid volume pumped with losses in whole blood, plasma, and total extracellular fluid; and (3) *Capacitance shock:* a decrease in the vascular bed tone generally induced by one of two pathophysiologic states: (a) loss of neurologic homeostasis secondary to spinal injury; or (b) sepsis or secondary metabolic influences causing a direct effect on peripheral resistance, venous capacitance, and possible opening of peripheral AV shunts. Although massive trauma may induce a shock state involving any or all of the above-listed mechanisms, the use of massive fluid replacement acutely is most commonly necessitated by the hypovolemic state.

This chapter presents a discussion of the pathophysiologic fluid shifts induced by large volume losses, and a rational means for correction of the deficit. Although it is commonly agreed that volume restoration is by necessity the priority of shock management, the most physiologic method for replacing and possibly retarding further fluid shifts is still debated. Therefore, we will define and attempt to establish with experimental and clinical data an approach which we feel is most appropriate for the treatment of the hypovolemic state subsequent to massive trauma.

Intravascular fluid losses secondary to massive trauma occur owing to two basic mechanisms. In one, there is an obvious disruption of continuity of the vascular tree with rapid egress of intravascular volume. It occurs subsequent to either penetrating or blunt trauma, and loss of volume continues until either spasm or external compression, that is, tamponade or mechanical compression (e.g., a hemostat), causes flow within the vessel to cease. Loss of intravascular volume also occurs subsequent to changes induced in the endothelial lining of the vascular tree, allowing intravascular fluid to leak into the extravascular space. This second type of loss can be induced by myriad causes, including direct vascular damage from intraoperative exposure of peritoneal surfaces, burn injuries, or massive soft tissue crush injuries. In addition, many other pathophysiologic events have been postulated as capable of inducing an endothelial cell leakiness, although the exact mechanisms involved are still not known. Incriminated are the activation of kinins; release of histamine from mast cells; activation of the complement cascade with subsequent release of anaphylactoxins; aggregation of both platelets and neutrophils with subsequent plugging of the microcirculation, degranulation, and vascular injury; prostaglandin synthesis and release at multicellular sites inducing endothelial leakiness; and direct endothelial cell injury subsequent to anoxic insult. Regardless of the etiology, the result is an obligate loss of volume from the intravascular space into surrounding tissues.

What is seen clinically is the physiologic response of the patient to this decrease in intravascular volume. Arterial blood pressure is determined by the cardiac output and the peripheral vascular resistance. When the cardiac output is reduced because of loss of intravascular volume, the blood pressure will remain normal only so long as an increased peripheral vascular resistance can compensate for this reduction in output (which is normally up to 20 percent of the intravascular volume).[4] The result of a fall in intravascular volume is stimulation of the sympathetic nervous system and adrenal medulla with a simultaneous inhibition of the vagal-medullary center. Consequently, there is an increase in heart rate to help compensate for the reduction in blood volume, and concomitantly, total peripheral resistance can double in response to hypovolemia-induced catecholamine release. The increase in vascular resistance is variable, depending upon the organ system studied. While the heart and brain maintain perfusion, other organ systems demonstrate a marked decrease in perfusion. Clinically, the dermis and the kidneys demonstrate decreased perfusion with cool, dusky skin and oliguria, as the host attempts to increase intravascular volume and core perfusion. This physiologic response is augmented by the endocrine release of antidiuretic hormone, aldosterone, and corticosteroids, which supplement peripheral resistance by further decreasing flow to muscles, gut, liver, spleen, and kidneys. During mild to moderate hypovolemia (i.e., 20 to 30 percent of intravascular volume) the mean arterial pressure (MAP) is maintained at the expense of cardiac output (CO). However, cellular perfusion to vital organs is not depressed to injurious levels. With larger losses of intravascular volume, MAP cannot be maintained and resultant hypotension produces the cellular insult seen in hypovolemic shock.[4]

RATIONALE FOR CHOICE OF RESUSCITATIVE FLUID

In current treatment of hypovolemic shock, two asanguinous fluids are commonly used to restore circulatory volume in addition to replacement with blood. These resuscitative fluids are balanced salt solutions (BSS, usually Ringer's lactate) or a 5 percent albumin solution in Ringer's lactate. Theoretically, the primary difference between these two solutions is the colloidal osmotic pressure of the albumin solution.[5] Numerous arguments have evolved in support of one or the other over the recent years. Support for using BSS involves primarily: (1) during shock, an obligate loss of isotonic fluid occurs from the extracellular space—this deficiency is better replaced by a fluid which rapidly equilibrates with the extracellular space;[3,6-10] (2) no evidence exists of an increased morbidity or mortality secondary to the appropriate use of BSS;[11-14] and (3) there is no increased incidence of pulmonary edema in patients resuscitated with BSS and a probable decrease in renal complications.[15-19] In favor of the use of albumin solutions for resuscitation are: (1) the oncotic solution is retained in the intravascular space longer (as predicted by Starling's Law),[20] thus decreasing the amount of resuscitative fluid volume required; (2) the decreased loss of fluid from the intravascular space may help protect against the development of postresuscitative pulmonary edema;[21,22] and (3) the hypo-oncotic condition commonly noted in the immediate postresuscitative period is corrected, and theoretically, should "pull" sequestered fluid from the interstitial into the intravascular space.[5,21-23] These points will now be discussed in more detail.

Extracellular Fluid Changes

Shires and associates developed a method to simultaneously measure red blood cell mass total volume using ^{51}Cr-tagged red blood cells, total plasma volume using ^{131}I- and ^{125}I-tagged human serum albumin, and total body extracellular fluid volume by using ^{35}S-labeled sodium sulfate.[24] Following intravenous injection, each of the isotopes can be measured after equilibrium is achieved, and the total volumes into which each of the isotopes have been distributed can be determined by dilution principles using multiple sampling techniques. In animals bled 10 percent of whole blood volume, measurement of fluid losses using the triple isotope technique demonstrated that the decrease in the extracellular fluid volume was equal to, and only to, that lost as plasma volume during hemorrhage.[3] Using the same model, studies were done with increasing but still sublethal hemorrhages of 25 to 50 percent of the measured blood volume. Again, the loss of red cell mass and plasma were confirmed using the above techniques; however, in addition, it was noted that the functional extracellular fluid volume (sulfate space) was decreased in excess of the measured plasma loss. Since there was no obvious external loss as measured by ^{35}S distribution, it was postulated that the reduction was secondary to internal redistribution of the extracellular fluid.[8] These animals were different from the initial group in that all had been subjected to a period of induced hypotension in addition to a pure mechanical blood loss. In additional studies, dogs were subjected to an established lethal period of shock by removing a sufficient blood volume, and then were subsequently reinfused with all shed blood. Measurements revealed that the red blood cell mass and plasma volume returned to baseline levels; however, again there remained a deficit in the functional extracellular fluid volume. If resuscitation consisted of both return of shed blood plus additional plasma replacement, there was again a return of blood volume to normal; however, a decrease in extracellular fluid volume remained. In contrast, dogs of comparable degree and duration of shock treated with an extracellular-type fluid (such as a BSS) plus return of shed blood had not only blood volume return to normal, but also exhibited a normal functional extracellular fluid volume. Dogs with induced hemorrhagic shock producing an LD_{80} when resuscitated with shed blood only, had a mortality of 70 percent when plasma, in addition to whole blood, was used for resuscitation. Animals treated with lactated Ringer's solution plus shed blood had a mortality of 30 percent.[7]

Using volume distribution curves for ^{35}S in sustained, untreated hemorrhagic shock animals, there is a measured reduction in the total extracellular fluid (i.e., late equilibrated volume of the radiosulfate) when compared with the preshock volumes. At all levels of induced shock, even at very low levels, there is a reduction in the functional extracellular fluid volume (i.e., early equilibrated volume of ^{35}S). However, the total (late equilibrated) extracellular fluid volume may remain normal at low levels of induced shock, or after partial resuscitation of shock. Subsequent studies have confimed that if the hypotensive episode is not sufficient to produce a reduction in the total, measured extracellular fluid volume, the reduction may exist only in the functional extracellular fluid space.[9] If shock levels are minimal, and aggressive early resuscitation occurs rapidly, the results of ^{35}S measurements of extracellular volume must be interpreted with care because the total extracellular fluid volume and the early functional extracellular fluid deficit may not be measured correctly.[10]

The source of the interstitial volume loss during shock is not explained by an extra-anatomic loss. Although some transcapillary refilling of the intravascular space does occur in response to hemorrhage and shock, the response initially is limited, and the total reduction cannot be explained by the amount of fluid which is pulled into the intravascular space.[3] Thus, subsequent studies were done by Shires' group to evaluate the loss of the functional extracellular volume as an isotonic shift into the intracellular cell mass.

Skeletal muscle cells were studied to measure intracellular swelling in response to hemorrhagic shock. Ion transport across the cell membrane was measured by using an ultramicro-electrode to determine the transmembrane potential in vivo before and after hemorrhagic shock. These measurements revealed that in acute hemorrhagic shock skeletal muscle cells develop a constant and sustained reduction in the normal negative transmembrane potential.[25] The cell membrane sodium pump contributes to the normal membrane potential, and appears to be impaired in the above situation. Ischemia appears to be necessary to depress membrane sodium pump function since hemorrhage insufficient to produce hypotension does not depress the transmembrane potential. An ischemic etiology is further supported by modifying other variables such as pH, carbon dioxide tension (P_{CO_2}), and bicarbonate levels which do not influence the membrane potential.

Additional studies in the dog hemorrhagic shock model have contributed supportive evidence that the loss in transmembrane potential is related to a deficiency in sodium pump function.[26] Using microtechniques, the interstitial fluid of skeletal muscle can be directly aspirated in vivo. Aspirations before and during hemorrhagic shock reveal that while the plasma potassium levels rise only minimally during shock, the directly-aspirated interstitial fluid potassium reaches levels greater than 15 mEq per liter. This is compatible with a loss of intracellular potassium into the interstitial fluid while sodium, chloride and water content are passively sequestered intracellularly. Studies using primates subjected to hemorrhagic shock reveal a similar phenomenon and that the interstitial potassium levels are converted to normal following treatment with resuscitation to normotensive levels. Using the primate model, data has also been obtained on muscle biopsies during shock which show an increase in sodium and water content intracellularly and a loss of potassium.[3]

In shocked primates, skeletal muscle cells isolated in vitro not only show a loss in the myocyte cellular membrane potential, but also both a decrease in the amplitude of the action potential and a prolongation of repolarization and depolarization times.[25] Resuscitation reverses these changes with the re-establishment of normal transmembrane potentials. However, there is a delay in return to normal repolarization times which may remain prolonged for several days. The pathophysiologic process responsible for this may be either a membrane protein injury, which requires repair or may be secondary to a depletion of energy stores (i.e., adenosine triphosphate), which requires a more prolonged period to generate normal levels and restore normal repolarization times.

The data show that the decrease in functional extracellular fluid appears to be due in part to an isotonic sequestration within the skeletal muscle cell mass in response to shock injury. Additionally, other cell types have been shown to increase both in intracellular sodium and volume in response to shock states. Neurons in vitro have been shown to increase in intracellular volume similar to myocytes in response to hypovolemic shock. There is also an increase in the internal sodium content of red blood cells during severe hemorrhagic shock. Thus, many diverse cell types are capable of taking up extracellular fluid in response to shock injury.

A major acellular sump for both sodium and water during hemorrhagic shock is the interstitial ground substance and collagen. In vivo, after a hypotensive challenge, a significant increase in wet weight and uptake of previously injected radioactive sodium is noted in the rat tail, which is over 90 percent extracellular collagen.[27] Fulton[28] used subcutaneously placed dehydrated collagen strips in dogs to demonstrate that a systemic hypotensive insult produced in these collagen strips causes a significant increase in both water and sodium content compared with controls. Thus, not only does the intracellular volume of multiple cell types increase in response to hypotensive insult, but also the interstitial ground substance and extracellular collagen serve as sources for the uptake of significant amounts of both water and sodium. The result is the decrease in functional extracellular fluid volume described by Shires and associates. Further, the magnitude of the changes is directly related to both the severity and the duration of the hypotensive insult.

Several other investigators have substantiated the previous data using various animal models. Studies by Grayson, LoHete, and Moyer[29] approached the problem from another point of view and concluded that the total available body sodium content was, in fact, the most important factor in determining the final plasma volume. They did not believe that the oncotic pressure was paramount in controlling the plasma volume. They pointed out that even severe hypoalbuminemia was compatible with normal existence and a normal plasma volume. Using a dog model of progressive total body sodium loss, they demonstrated that the plasma volume fell while, in contrast, albumin concentration rose. They concluded that if the key to plasma volume was total sodium content rather than albumin levels, restoration of total plasma volume should be accomplished using BSS plus return of shed red blood cells. Similar to the work of Shires, they showed that dogs bled until respiratory arrest developed could be salvaged by replacement of blood volume plus infusion of electrolyte solution. The plasma volume also returned to normal in these animals. Experiments using resuscitation with shed blood alone or in combination with dextran, or 5 percent glucose led to a much lower survival rate (less than 40 percent). In contrast, resuscitation with blood plus Ringer's lactate led to a high survival rate (approximately 80 percent). Fulton, using a dialysis system to deplete sodium selectively in the dog, was able to produce a reduction in cardiac output, arterial blood pressure, urine volume, oxygen consumption, and plasma volume in lieu of overt volume changes.

Data obtained from the dog hemorrhagic shock model are debated, owing to the occurrence of both splanchnic and pulmonary congestion as well as endocrine changes in the dog which are not seen in the primate. Additional studies have been done by Eaton,[16] and Moss and associates[17,23] using primates rather than dogs in a hemorrhagic shock model. In these experiments, hemorrhage was induced to produce a 100 percent mortality if untreated. Treatment consisted of either electrolyte solution or 5 percent albumin in electrolyte solution, with or without return of shed blood. Fluid was induced at a rate and volume to restore normal hemodynamic values similar to the clinical setting. Using these criteria, the volume of electrolyte solution required for resuscitation was three times greater than that of colloid solution or blood. At completion of resuscitation, the hematocrit had returned to normal in all groups, with shed blood returned consistent with a restoration of a normal plasma volume. As expected, a drop in total plasma proteins was seen in the saline-treated group. However, other indices of normal circulation and perfusion were restored, including cardiac output, pulmonary vascular resistance, serum lactate levels, venous Po_2, and urine output.

In summary, there is a measurable reduction in the extravascular, extracellular fluid volume in response to hemorrhagic shock. Concomitantly, the cellular response to the hypotensive insult is demonstrated as a depression in the active transport of ions with an increased intracellular level of sodium, chloride, and water content with an increased extracellular level of potassium. As stated earlier, restoration of the depleted extracellular fluid is not only of significant benefit in the clinical situation, but also experimentally produces a normalization of potassium levels in the extracellular, interstitial fluid space and sodium and chloride levels intracellularly. This restoration can best be obtained by using a noncolloid isotonic saline solution which rapidly distributes within the total extracellular volume.

Pulmonary Consequences of Shock and Resuscitation

The major argument today is whether the use of BSS resuscitation leads to an increased incidence of acute respiratory distress syndrome in the clinical setting. The primary focus for the use of colloid resuscitation for trauma has revolved around the potential protective pulmonary effects achieved using colloid supplementation. An increase in plasma oncotic pressure should partially prevent loss of intravascular volume into the interstitial space, or conversely should facilitate the removal of excess fluid which is already present in the interstitium. This rationale is based upon a simplified closed system model of Starling's Law.[20,22] An assumption in the simplified Starling equation is that the capillaries have the ability to retain plasma proteins. The initial in vitro experiments were performed on isolated organ preparations which ignored the presence of lymph flow in vivo, thus artificially creating the closed system assumed in the simplified Starling Law.[30] In these preparations, large amounts of edema occur which are at least 10 times normal, diluting the interstitial protein and increasing interstitial pressure. This large increase in interstitial pressure causes a rapid equilibration of venous and extravascular pressures, preventing the normal venous leak and exchange of protein. In these in vitro preparations, hyperoncotic colloid solutions given intravascularly were demonstrated to pull fluid from the interstitium into the intravascular space.

Several investigators[22,31,32] have shown this not to be true in vivo with an active extravascular circulation of plasma proteins via the lymphatic system. The lymphatic system provides a route through which fluid can flow from the interstitium back into the blood. More important, the lymphatics also remove proteins from the interstitium. This maintains interstitial oncotic pressure near normal. If this mechanism were not present, the rising interstitial oncotic pressure would significantly alter capillary fluid flux and gross tissue edema would result. A continuous transcapillary escape of albumin has been measured at approximately 5 percent of the total pool per hour in normal adults. This approximately triples during albumin infusion (reviewed in reference 22). The safety factor present in all tissues against edema formation is increased lymph flow. Lymph flow has been known to increase 20 times normal before edema occurs.[5] Experimentally, the rapid loss of 30 percent of the total protein concentration of the circulation (which is consistent with the reduction in plasma proteins seen postresuscitation with BSS) can be compensated for by increased lymphatic drainage. Measurement of this venular leakage into the interstitium and separate lymphatic protein concentration measurements argue against the assumption that the nonprotein fluid in the interstitium is removed by oncotic pressures in the intravascular space.[31,32] In fact, in vivo, significant resorption of interstitial fluids into the vascular system has not been demonstrated.

The ability of different organ tissues to retain or leak plasma proteins through their capillary surfaces is quite variable. The lung appears to have one of the highest protein flux rates of any organ in the normal state, and demonstrates one of the greatest increases in tissue volume resulting from fluid accumulation under pathologic conditions.[5] Experimentally, tissues accumulating the largest volumes of interstitial fluid require the longest period of time to revert to a normal hydration state. Therefore, it is argued that patients who have lost large quantities of intravascular colloid and have had their intravascular volume restored with only crystalloid solutions will be more likely to develop acute respiratory distress syndrome. Maintenance of the plasma oncotic pressure should be important in decreasing the amount of the interstitial fluid accumulation by the lung and subsequently decreasing or ablating the onset of the acute respiratory distress syndrome.[5]

Logically, it could be argued that infusion of large volumes of electrolyte solution during resuscitation would favor development of generalized interstitial edema, and, in particular, a pathophysiologically significant pulmonary interstitial edema. Eaton,[16] in early studies on this problem, demonstrated that resuscitation in dogs using BSS as compared with plasma produced approximately a twofold increase in total lung water. Using a baboon hemorrhage model, lung water measurements have been repeated similar to the work of Eaton. Resuscitation of these animals using either 5 percent albumin or BSS at an approximate 1:3 volume ratio was used to measure the response in total lung water content. In these studies, resuscitation with either solution produced no significant differences in pulmonary water content between either of the groups or between each group and its respective control value.[17]

Are changes in pulmonary water content physiologically important? It is argued that although the total lung water content may not be increased with saline resuscitation, it is conceivable that there is pathophysiologic derangement of the tissue water distribution. Ultrastructure evaluation of the baboon lung following either a 5 percent albumin solution or saline resuscitation demonstrated no detectable difference between animals resuscitated with either solution.[17] There is no increase in the interstitial space or swelling of the collagen fibers in either group of animals. Moss and associates,[17] in another approach measured the effect of resuscitation on lung compliance. It was postulated that if pulmonary edema were developing, a stiffening of the lung should occur with a subsequent decrease in lung compliance. These investigators demonstrated that hemorrhage produces an acute increase in compliance due to a decrease in total lung fluid volume. Resuscitation with either an oncotic solution or BSS produces a decrease to baseline compliance which does not differ from control values.

Experimentally, it has not been possible to demonstrate that lung water can be decreased in vivo by raising the plasma oncotic pressure. Specifically, in regard to the pulmonary circulation, there is evidence suggesting that albumin and other plasma proteins enter and collect in the pulmonary interstitium freely, and that this process effectively limits the absorptive ability of the plasma oncotic pressure.[32] It is postulated that excess albumin therapy, and thus interstitial pooling, may actually aggravate rather than aid patients with pulmonary insufficiency.[33] Additionally, lymph flow rates seem to be inversely proportional to interstitial albumin concentration, so that again the albumin infusion tends to favor the accumulation of fluid in the interstitium. Rats loaded with concentrated albumin show a peak of pulmonary extravascular albumin at eight hours, persisting for at least 48 hours. In the critically ill patient, concentrated albumin therapy may be even more likely to sequester albumin into the interstitial spaces leading to interstitial edema and organ dysfunction.[33] The above data further support the use of a BSS rather than colloid solutions for resuscitation of hypovolemic shock. The use of BSS does not lead to an increase in pulmonary interstitial fluid and prevents the potential increase induced by resuscitation with colloid solutions.

Renal Responses

Turning to the renal response, the data suggest that renal function is less effectively restored in patients resuscitated with 5 percent albumin solution. Experimentally, Moss's group[23] used awake, nonheparinized baboons in a hemorrhagic shock model. The baboons were randomly selected, after an induced hemorrhagic shock period of 60 minutes, for resuscitation with either Ringer's lactate and shed red cells, or with a 5 percent albumin solution plus shed red cells. Resuscitation was sufficient to restore cardiovascular variables to baseline. In the Ringer's lactate group a return of urine output to normal levels was recorded within 30 minutes of the initial resuscitation, with return to normal electrolyte balance and normal renal tubular function judged by the rate of p-aminohippuric acid (PAH) renal extraction. The group contrasted this response to animals resuscitated with 5 percent albumin solution and demonstrated a slower return of basal urine outputs, an increased intravascular volume, an increase in plasma osmolarity and an increase in intravascular sodium concentration. There was also a depressed renal tubular absorption of both sodium and potassium with an inappropriate increase in free water, despite the increased osmolarity of the intravascular fluid, coupled with a significant reduction in the clearance ratio of PAH. The group concluded that the resuscitation of hemorrhagic shock with BSS in conjunction with red cell replacement is not only equal to, but much more effective than, resuscitation with colloid solution for restoration of normal renal tubular function.

Other Considerations

A theoretic point of concern is the effect of albumin solutions on hepatic function. The level of hepatic interstitial albumin appears to play a critical role in the control of albumin synthesis as a feedback mechanism.[34] An increase in hepatic interstitial albumin, as has been demonstrated secondary to albumin fluid therapy, depresses the endogenous hepatic production of albumin. Whereas a decrease in albumin levels after BSS resuscitation should stimulate albumin production.

Finally, from a point of cost-effectiveness, a bottle of saline costs only one-fiftieth of an equal volume of 5 percent albumin.[17] Even if resuscitation using BSS requires an increased volume compared with albumin solution, the cost of using albumin still greatly exceeds that of BSS. If a colloid solution is experimentally and clinically no better than an electrolyte solution for resuscitation of shock, the expense alone makes the BSS preferable.

Clinical Studies

There have been few good clinical trials directed at comparing BSS versus albumin resuscitation, owing to the complexity of the problem. Carey and associates[11] performed a good clinical study of the treatment of traumatic shock in a group of injured patients in Vietnam. Fifty-six massively injured patients were treated with BSS plus whole blood. Patients were treated to restore hemodynamic variables to baseline. The patients were given an average of 12 liters of electrolyte solution and 5 liters of blood during the first 24 hours and responded with a good clinical course and no evidence of pulmonary edema.

Additionally, 10 similar patients were treated with a 5 percent albumin solution plus whole blood, and although all survived, they responded less well clinically and required twice as much blood and produced half as much urine as those receiving Ringer's lactate.

Two often quoted clinical trials involve two groups of patients who were studied during elective abdominal vascular procedures. The first of these, by Skillman and associates,[21] involved randomized treatment of 16 patients, who received either an albumin or a sodium-rich, intraoperative fluid regimen. Plasma volume, oncotic pressure, alveolar to arterial oxygen tension differences, creatinine clearance, body weight, and fluid and sodium intake were studied preoperatively and postoperatively. Postoperatively, the albumin resuscitated group had a significantly greater circulating albumin mass and intravascular oncotic pressure than the electrolyte resuscitated group. Most significantly, an increase in pulmonary alveolar-arterial oxygen difference $P(A-a)O_2$ and expansion of the extracellular fluid volume was measured in the electrolyte-solution-treated group compared with the albumin-resuscitated group. There was no apparent adverse effect on creatinine clearance in the albumin-treated group compared with the electrolyte group.

The second study, by Virgilio and associates,[13] evaluated 29 patients undergoing elective abdominal aortic surgery. Again, multiple variables were randomly studied, particularly pertaining to pulmonary function. The patients were randomly resuscitated with either Ringer's lactate or with a 5 percent albumin solution with blood loss replaced as packed red blood cells. Again, they showed a much larger requirement for fluid in the electrolyte resuscitated group, with a concomitant decrease in the intravascular oncotic pressure. However, in comparison with the previous study, they noticed that although a slight increase in pulmonary shunt fraction occurred in both groups following operation, there was no difference between the two groups. Further, fluid balance, total fluid infused, sodium balance, total sodium infused, intravascular oncotic pressure, and the gradient between intravascular oncotic pressure and pulmonary wedge pressure did not correlate with the pulmonary shunt value. In this study, two patients in the albumin-resuscitated group experienced pulmonary edema; whereas in the Ringer's lactate-resuscitated group, there were no cases of pulmonary edema. These authors concluded that there was no evidence to support maintaining the intravascular pulmonary oncotic pressure by using protein containing solutions; and that if titrated to physiologic end-points (e.g., maintenance of normal filling pressures), even the increased volume of BSS required was well tolerated. Important in the evaluation of these two studies is that in the Skillman study, even though a larger fluid load was given to the electrolyte-resuscitated group, the patients in this group had a postoperative plasma volume significantly lower than the preoperative value. In the second study, patients resuscitated with the electrolyte solution received adequate resuscitation to maintain normal plasma volumes. As noted above, a decrease in plasma volume and interstitial fluid volume may well contribute to cellular injury and to the increased $P(A-a)O_2$ seen in the first study. Additionally, calculations of pulmonary gas exchange in under-resuscitated patients (i.e., decreased CO and mixed venous oxygen tension), resulted in an increased $P(A-a)O_2$ which was not related to pulmonary edema. Also, the creatinine clearance functions between the two groups were not comparable since clearance preoperatively in the albumin group was only 50 percent of that of the electrolyte group. It should be noted that since both groups were elective, non-shocked patients with normal capillary endothelial membrane barriers, maintenance of adequate intravascular volume would be expected to have no variable effect on pulmonary function in the two groups studied.

Lowe and coworkers[12] and Moss and associates[14] have extended these findings in two groups of trauma patients. In the first, 141 patients undergoing laparotomy for trauma were selected randomly for resuscitation either with washed red cells plus Ringer's lactate or with Ringer's lactate plus albumin. Hemodynamic variables were stabilized. In this study, it was noted that the albumin-resuscitated patients required greater total volumes (5.9 versus 5.4 liters). Multiple pulmonary variables were followed for five days postoperatively pulmonary function tests (PFT), arterial blood gases (ABG), dead space/tidal volume [V_D/V_T], $P(A-a)O_2$, and intrapulmonary shunt). The overall results demonstrated no significant differences in survival rate, incidence of pulmonary failure, or postoperative pulmonary functions. However, the majority of these patients were not in shock, and again it could be argued that both groups should demonstrate minimal pulmonary pathology. Therefore, in a recent second study[14] trauma patients in shock undergoing laparotomy were studied in a similar fashion. Injuries and other criteria were comparable in the two groups. The results from this group of patients confirm the lack of differences in pulmonary function between the two resuscitation protocols.

In a clinical trial, Irwin and associates,[15] evaluated renal responses by randomly assigning patients undergoing elective intestinal surgery either to resuscitation with BSS or to a salt-restricted regimen. Patients treated with a restricted resuscitation had marked deficits in plasma volume postoperatively and an associated marked antidiuresis and decreases in renal function. In contrast, renal function was returned to normal by maintaining normal hemodynamic values using BSS resuscitation. Ledgerwood and Lucas[35] further demonstrated that resuscitation using an albumin solution in trauma patients not only failed to prevent weight gain and extracellular fluid loss during resuscitation, but was associated with a prolonged resuscitation phase and an increased need for both blood and saline resuscitation. These patients also had lower hourly urine volumes, and the authors suggest that albumin may interfere with the saline diuresis commonly seen during resuscitation and prolong the renal function decrement of the hypovolemic state.

A concluding point to be considered in the use of albumin solutions for hypovolemic resuscitation has been reported by Kovalick and associates.[36] In their series of trauma patients, the use of albumin in resuscitation produced normal serum albumin levels and higher total calcium levels, but significantly decreased the free calcium level and calcium to total calcium ratio. The level of calcium and calcium to total calcium ratio correlated directly with the calculated heart work unit index in both albumin and BSS patients. Thus, while raising the total calcium, albumin binds serum calcium and depresses myocardial function. This dysfunction appears to be partially responsible for the heart failure and pulmonary edema seen in some albumin-resuscitated patients. Overall, if adequate hemodynamic monitoring is used in conjunction with restoration of intravascular and total extracellular volume, we believe that BSS is preferable to colloid solution as an *adjunct* to blood replacement in the management of patients with massive trauma.

SPECIFIC CHOICES FOR RESUSCITATION FLUID

Electrolyte Solutions

The issue of which electrolyte solution is preferable, that is, normal saline or Ringer's lactate, should be addressed. Theoretically, these two solutions should affect the acid-base status of the patient quite differently. This question was addressed by Corgan and associates,[37] using a hemorrhagic shock model in mongrel dogs. The dogs were treated normal saline or Ringer's solution subsequent to a 1000 ml blood loss. All dogs survived, and most variables did not differ significantly. During resuscitation, there was no difference between groups as heart rates returned toward normal, cardiac output increased, arterial P_{CO_2} and serum potassium remained unchanged, and the blood lactate levels decreased. The one variable which did remain separate in the two groups throughout the resuscitation period was the blood pH, which initially dropped and then rose toward normal. Overall, the change in pH from the end of the shock period to the end of resuscitation in the Ringer's lactate group showed a net gain of 0.09 pH unit, while the saline-treated group had a net loss of 0.04 pH unit. These data are consistent with other experimental studies using Ringer's lactate, which have shown that Ringer's lactate plus whole blood resuscitation returns the arterial pH to normal.

The pH of the solutions are 6.1 for normal saline and 6.5 for Ringer's lactate, which has a lactate content of 28 mEq per liter. Theoretically, if the L-lactate was completely metabolized to bicarbonate, the pH of the Ringer's lactate-treated group should be much higher. Failure of this to occur is likely owing to impaired metabolism in the liver subsequent to the hypotensive insult with decreased perfusion. Finally, it should be noted that in both groups the arterial lactate levels remained above normal, but the final lactate levels were identical. The level of resuscitation was therefore considered equal between the two groups, and the difference in the pH was secondary to increased bicarbonate from metabolized lactate. Although addition of blood to the resuscitation provides the buffer necessary to restore a normal pH, theoretically it is appealing to use a solution which most rapidly and efficiently corrects the acidosis induced by hypotensive shock. Ringer's lactate appears to be preferable over the use of normal saline in the initial resuscitation of the hypotensive patient.[37]

Blood Substitutes

Debate also exists over the use of other blood substitutes in place of blood, or when blood is not available. The most commonly used substitute is human plasma. However, plasma carries with it the same risk of viral hepatitis as whole blood, and pooled plasma carries an even greater risk. There is also risk of a poorly understood antigen-antibody reaction occurring with homologous plasma. Finally, the volume of plasma required for resuscitation is large, and restoration of blood volume is not generally feasible with plasma alone because of rapid incorporation into the extracellular fluid volume and the limited oxygen carrying capacity compared with red blood cells. Thus, plasma or albumin is a transient blood volume substitute at best. If blood is truly not available and none is anticipated for some length of time, the use of plasma or 5 percent albumin solution as a stopgap measure is reasonable *after* replacement of the ECF deficit with electrolyte solutions. Dextran has been advocated as a replacement of the intravascular volume, but has no oxygen carrying capacity, and like other plasma substitutes, has an established incidence of anaphylactoid reactions. High molecular weight dextran has also been shown to produce defects in the clotting mechanism which, in the normal volunteer, occur after infusion of more than one liter of dextran. Low molecular weight dextran in the range of 35,000–40,000 has been advocated because of its ability to lower blood viscosity, and thus prevent agglutination and sludging in the microcirculation during the low-flow state induced by hypovolemic shock.[38] However, Replogle, Jundsler, and Gross[39] have shown that the effect of the low molecular weight dextran on viscosity is produced by hemodilution, or change in blood volume; and that when these variables are controlled, there is no evidence for alteration of blood viscosity per se. Hydroxyethyl starch (HES) has been proposed as a nontoxic plasma expander with hemodynamic effects similar to other colloids. HES is nonallergic and produces less coagulopathy than dextran.[40] However, since its introduction in 1963, HES has not been shown to be superior to crystalloid for resuscitation and, as an artificial particulate, has the theoretic disadvantage of potentially depressing the reticuloendothelial system through a blockade effect.

THERAPY IN HYPOVOLEMIC SHOCK

Principles

As described above, the etiology of shock can be dependent on distinctly different mechanisms. The patient must be supported while the specific etiologic pathophysiology is diagnosed. Obviously, diagnosis will dictate the best course of treatment for the hypotensive state. As stated previously, the etiologies of shock can be loosely grouped into three main categories: (1) hypovolemic shock; (2) cardiogenic shock; and (3) shock induced by loss of peripheral resistance and increase in capacitance of vessels (i.e., neurogenic or septic shock). In the massively traumatized patient it is certainly possible for more than one etiologic factor to be present. However, for the purpose of this discussion, and owing to overwhelming preponderance as an etiologic agent, this discussion will be limited to resuscitation for hypovolemic shock.

In any massively traumatized patient, the initial step in evaluation and treatment is maintenance of an adequate airway and ventilatory status. If excessive external blood loss is occurring, then control should be achieved immediately and intravenous fluid therapy begun. Shortly after injury, extracellular fluid deficits secondary to extensive soft tissue crush injuries, burns, fractures, retroperitoneal, and intraperitoneal injuries frequently coexist with hemorrhagic (or external losses) shock. Significant internal redistribution of extracellular fluid may result from isotonic shifts of fluid which produce no measureable change in intravascular electrolyte patterns.[3] Additionally, functional extracellular losses are very difficult to estimate (e.g., the peritoneum has the same surface area as the skin and can sequester several liters of fluid). With both rapid extra-anatomic blood loss and reduction in extracellular fluid secondary to massive trauma producing hypotension, the initial therapy started should be BSS. The use of plasma or other sources of protein are only rarely required (see discussion above).

The present treatment of hypovolemic shock is adequate replacement of the fluid lost. In the case of hemorrhagic shock, the fluid lost is blood and should be replaced with blood as soon as feasible. The use of properly crossmatched type-specific whole blood is still the primary therapy. When crossmatched blood of the proper type is not immediately available, type-specific or Rh-negative donor group O blood with low anti-A titer can be administered. In addition, however, because of changes induced in the intravascular and interstitial fluid volumes by the hypotensive insult, an effective resuscitative regimen should also include additional replacement using BSS.

Therapeutic Approach

Following is a proposal which has been used successfully as an effective therapeutic regimen for the treatment of hypovolemic shock. The traumatized patient is initially resuscitated with an infusion of lactated Ringer's solution through large bore upper extremity catheters. Simultaneously, blood is drawn for type and crossmatch. The rate of infusion is rapid, so that within the initial 45–60 minutes at least 1000 to 2000 ml of lactated Ringer's solution can be given intravenously. The rationale behind this approach is as follows: The infusion is a trial to help determine the amount of blood loss present, or the presence of continuing active blood loss. Experimentally, if the infusion of 1 to 2 liters of BSS restores a previously hypotensive patient to a normotensive state, the blood loss existing at the time of admission was minimal. If there is no ongoing blood loss, the hypotensive episode can be controlled by infusion of the BSS alone. However, if blood loss is severe or hemorrhage is continuing, the blood pressure response and the decrease in pulse rate seen with the rapid infusion of lactated Ringer's solution will be transient. If this occurs, the patient needs to receive blood which has been typed and crossmatched and is now available. By definition, the lack of sustained response to the BSS infusion necessitates the addition of blood and dictates against increasing BSS replacement alone. The use of the BSS allows time for the accurate typing and crossmatching of the blood. Experimental data (see above) also demonstrate that the restoration of the depleted extravascular fluid volume is beneficial in decreasing both the morbidity and mortality of the hypotensive insult.

The primary treatment for hemorrhagic shock is replacement with blood. However, several facets of stored bank blood use should be recognized. Blood stored in acid-citrate-dextrose (ACD) solution for up to three weeks produces survival of at least 70 percent of its cells in the recipient during this period. However, stored blood demonstrates a rapid decline in 2,3-diphosphoglycerate (2,3-DPG) and thus a progressive increase in hemoglobin-oxygen affinity (left shift of the oxygen dissociation curve) occurs. Although the 2,3-DPG can be restored to normal levels in vivo, this requires at least 24 hours following transfusion. Immediately after transfusion, oxygen delivery may be impaired by the administration of large amounts of banked blood. To compensate for this deficit, the age of all transfused blood should be recorded, and if there is a significant amount of blood older than several days, attempts should be instituted to obtain fresh whole blood for additional transfusion. This problem is reduced by use of citrate-phosphate-dextrose (CPD), available in many blood banks.

Evaluation of Patient Response

If the patient fails to respond to the management program outlined, other causes of shock must be evaluated and corrected. The possible causes are multiple: (1) continuing blood loss from the primary injury or from a source not initially considered; (2) inadequate replacement of fluids; (3) indirect consequences of massive trauma, such as cardiac tamponade, or tension pneumothorax, or both, and (4) myocardial failure either as a result of inadequate perfusion during shock or secondary to underlying cardiac disease. Resolution of this problem requires careful clinical evaluation of the patient and measurement of several hemodynamic variables which are readily available in emergency situations.

Hemodynamically, (1) an estimate of the amount of fluid present in the intravascular system and (2) the capacity of the myocardium to circulate this fluid should be evaluated. A direct measurement of the intravascular volume would be the ideal approach, but is currently impractical. Attempts to measure blood volume have proven to be very erratic and unreliable during acute hemorrhagic shock state.[41] Similarly, determination of the size of the extracellular fluid volume would be useful. However, this is largely a research tool which has not been applicable in the acute clinical situation. Central venous pressure (CVP) measurement is currently used as the most easily applied clinical measurement for estimating the balance between volume of the intravascular space and myocardial function.[41] The CVP monitor has been popularized as a reliable method to obtain an approximation of the adequacy of the circulatory status to maintain normal venous return to the heart. As a one-time measurement, the central venous pressure must be used cautiously and in conjunction with other measurements and observations. When the CVP is used as a serial test, important information can be derived from the response to rapid administration of fluid challenges. The ability of the myocardium to maintain adequate circulation also needs to be assessed. This is usually accomplished by determination of arterial blood pressure, either direct or indirect.

Through use of these simple hemodynamic monitors, the relative volume status of the complicated trauma patient can often be rapidly determined, and appropriate volume replacement performed. A depressed or normal central venous pressure that does not rise in response to BSS is usually indicative of continued hypovolemia and requires further fluid resuscitation. Correction is indicated by a gradual increase in both CVP and arterial pressure. A minimal or transient rise in blood pressure and CVP is indicative of continued volume loss, most likely secondary to bleeding. In contrast, the presence of an elevated central venous pressure rising rapidly with the administration of fluids, which produces either no change or a decrease in perfusion, is strongly suggestive of an impairment in myocardial pumping ability. Appropriate myocardial support should be given. However, a decreased myocardial contractility secondary to mechanical obstruction must be ruled out. Such causes should be considered as cardiac tamponade or mediastinal compression secondary to tension pneumothorax or hemothorax. The potential for such occult problems in the patient with multiple injuries must always be of concern.

Above all, it must be remembered that the ultimate criterion of adequate response to treatment of hypovolemia is response of the patient. Two prime indicators of adequate resuscitation and perfusion are restoration of normal cerebration and adequate urine output. Also of use, but more difficult to measure, are signs of increased dermal perfusion. If an inadequate response is noted, several aspects of care need to be considered. First is a search for continued bleeding from previously noted injuries or from sites which were initially not observed. The primary cause of the hypotensive state should be carefully re-evaluated to insure that it is no longer contributing. Special attention must also be paid to the basics of resuscitation. In particular, maintenance of adequate ventilation, control of the airway, and institution of assisted respiratory support, as necessary, may be indicated. Acceptable urine volume relies on restoration of adequate renal blood flow, not on the induction of an artificial diuresis. Use of osmotic diuretics or other diuretics, such as furosemide, in the presence of uncorrected intravascular volume will produce "urine for urine's sake," but has no physiologic basis for protection of renal function. It is, in fact, detrimental owing to further depletion of the intravascular and extravascular fluid volume, and subjects the kidneys to further insult secondary to decreased renal blood flow.

Finally, in the complex patient, more sophisticated hemodynamic monitoring can be usefully employed. Such measurements include cardiac output, peripheral resistance, and pulmonary artery and pulmonary artery wedge pressures (i.e., left atrial pressure), using the balloon tiped Swan-Ganz catheter.

Arguments against the use of CVP measurements in a complicated patient have been raised primarily because left ventricular overload and pulmonary edema can occur while right ventricular function remains adequate. This combination maintains normal central venous pressure. This can be seen after traumatic myocardial injury. The error can be partially eliminated by decreasing reliance solely on static CVP values and noting the response of myocardial pressures to fluid challenges as discussed previously. However, if concern persists, interpretation of myocardial function can be augmented by the measurement of pulmonary artery pressure and pulmonary wedge pressure, using the Swan-Ganz catheter in the pulmonary artery outflow track. Cardiac output can be estimated by using the arteriovenous oxygen gradient. However, this is erratic and unreliable in acute hemorrhagic states, and more direct measurements of cardiac output by dye or temperature dilution techniques are readily available via the Swan-Ganz catheter. By use of dilution techniques, cardiac output can be determined rapidly, accurately, and sequentially.

Using cardiac output and mean arterial pressure data, total systemic resistance can be calculated for evaluation. With normal or increased central venous pressure, and normal or high cardiac output simultaneous with persistent hypotension, the most likely cause is loss of peripheral vascular resistance. Decreased peripheral vascular resistance is rarely, if ever, seen in oligemic shock. It is most commonly due either to sepsis or neurogenic etiologies. In contrast, a high peripheral resistance, seen in hypovolemic shock with concomitant myocardial inefficiency can be reduced to increase cardiac output. However, before giving drugs to decrease systemic vascular resistance, insure that adequate volume has been replaced. There is little indication for use of vasopressors in hypovolemic shock.[42] Finally, a careful search should be instituted for primary or secondary metabolic abnormalities.

Postresuscitation Hypertension

The phenomenon of postresuscitation hypertension has recently been discussed. Ledgerwood and Lucas[35] reported frequent hypertension following successful resuscitation of severely injured patients with shock. The diagnosis is made by systolic and diastolic hypertension (greater than 150 to 100 mmHg) sustained for periods of at least six hours following successful resuscitation. It appears to be commonly associated with the most severely injured patients, and is associated with respiratory failure, hematuria, and central nervous system problems. The etiology of the postresuscitation hypertension appears to be secondary to a rapid intravascular influx of extracellular fluid which was sequestered during the obligate loss induced by hypotension. The extent of the extracellular obligate loss is directly related to the degree of cellular injury, and therefore, the duration and severity of the hypotensive insult. The hypothesis that administration of plasma, albumin, or diuretics, or a combination of them, during resuscitation can decrease fluid requirements has been advocated to decrease the degree of postresuscitation hypertension. However, in recent studies,[11,35] albumin not only failed to prevent weight gain and interstitial expansion, but was associated with needs for larger volumes of blood and saline and a more sustained postresuscitation hypertension. As noted above, the use of albumin was also associated with a lower urine output. This suggests that albumin may interfere with the saline diuresis seen postresuscitation, prolonging renal insufficiency by maintaining intravascular volume at the expense of interstitial fluid volume. This insult then inhibits ability of the kidneys to excrete the increased volume seen during mobilization of the extravascular fluid.

Because postresuscitative hypertension and increased morbidity are associated, attempts at prevention would seem beneficial. Respiratory failure was more common near the end of the resuscitative phase, was maximum at the peak of hypertension, and appeared to improve with diuresis. The difficulty is that there is no satisfactory method of determining the point at which the obligatory extracellular loss has been completed. This point in resuscitation can be identified partially by the need for smaller volumes of fluid to maintain blood pressure, urine output, and stable central venous pressure. If the patient becomes hypertensive or oliguric after the extracellular requirements have been met, diuretics should probably be used sparingly to facilitate sodium and water excretion. On those rare occasions when diuretics are indicated, care should be exercised to prevent overdiuresis due to the inability of the intravascular space to rapidly compensate for volume losses. It appears that the renal cellular damage initially induced by the hypotensive insult recovers at a slower rate than the rate of autoinfusion with mobilization of sequestered extravascular fluid. If use of diuretics fails to correct the hypertension, vasodilators should be considered to expand vascular capacitance and to allow the renal cellular dysfunction to recover. Once the kidneys can handle the increased volume load, the hypertension resolves spontaneously and is no longer a problem. This phenomenon again argues strongly for the rapid initial resuscitation of the hypotensive patient with maximal replacement of both intravascular and total extracellular fluid volumes, using both blood and BSS to efficiently restore cellular perfusion and prevent ongoing cellular damage.

REFERENCES

1. GROSS, SG: *A System of Surgery: Pathological, Diagnostic, Therapeutic and Operative,* Lea & Febiger, Philadelphia, 1872.
2. BLALOCK, A: *Principles of Surgical Care, Shock and Other Problems.* CV Mosby, St. Louis, 1940.

3. SHIRES, GT: *Principles and Management of Hemorrhagic Shock,* in SHIRES, GT (ED): *Care of the Trauma Patient,* ed 2. McGraw-Hill, New York, 1979, p 3.
4. LUCAS, CE: *Resuscitation of the injured patient: The three phases of treatment.* Surg Clin North Am 57:3, 1977.
5. GRANGER, DN, ET AL: *Physiologic basis for the clinical use of albumin solutions.* Surgeon General's Office, 146:97, 1978.
6. MOYER, CA, MORGRAF, HW, AND MONAFO, WW: *Burn shock and extravascular sodium deficiency—treatment with Ringer's solution with lactate.* Arch Surg 90:799, 1965.
7. SHIRES, GT, CARRICO, CJ, AND CANIZARO, PL: *Shock.* Philadelphia, WB Saunders, 1973, p 57.
8. SHIRES, GT, ET AL: *Fluid therapy in hemorrhagic shock.* Arch Surg 88:688, 1964.
9. CANIZARO, PC AND SHIRES, GT: *Fluid resuscitation in injured patients.* Surg Clin North Am 53:1341, 1973.
10. CARRICO, CJ, CANIZARO, PC, AND SHIRES, GT: *Fluid resuscitation following injury: Rationale for the use of balanced salt solutions.* Crit Care Med 4:46, 1976.
11. CAREY, LC, LOWREY, BD, AND CLOUTDIER, CT: *Hemorrhagic shock.* Curr Probl Surg 8:31, Jan, 1971.
12. LOWE, RJ, ET AL: *Crystolloid vs. colloid in the etiology of pulmonary failure after trauma: A randomized trial in man.* Surgery 81:676, 1977.
13. VIRGILIO, RW, ET AL: *Crystalloid vs. colloid resuscitation: Is one better? A randomized clinical study.* Surgery 85:129, 1979.
14. MOSS, GS, ET AL: *Colloid or crystalloid in the resuscitation of hemorrhagic shock: A controlled clinical trial.* Surgery 89:434, 1981.
15. IRWIN, TT, ET AL: *Plasma-volume deficits and salt and water excretion after surgery.* Lancet 2:1159, 1972.
16. EATON, RM: *Pulmonary edema.* J Thorac Surg 16:668, 1945.
17. MOSS, GS, ET AL: *Hemorrhagic shock in the baboon II. Changes in lung compliance associated with hemorrhagic shock and resuscitation.* J Trauma 8:842, 1968.
18. MOSS, GS: *An argument in favor of electrolyte solution for early resuscitation.* Surg Clin North Am 52:3, 1972.
19. SIEGEL, DC, ET AL: *Effects of saline and colloid resuscitation on renal function.* Ann Surg 177:51, 1973.
20. STARLING, EH: *On absorption of fluids from the connective tissue spaces.* J Physiol 19:312, 1895.
21. SKILLMAN, JJ, RESTALL, DS, AND SALZMAN, EW: *Randomized trial of albumin vs. electrolyte solutions during abdominal aortic operations.* Surgery 78:291, 1975.

22. MARTY, AT: *Hyperoncotic albumin therapy.* Surgeon General's Office 139:105, 1974.
23. MOSS, GS, ET AL: *Hemorrhagic shock in the baboon I. Circulatory and metabolic effects of dilutional therapy: preliminary report.* J Trauma 8:837, 1968.
24. SHIRES, GT, WILLIAMS, J, AND BROWN, FJ: *A method for simultaneous measurement of plasma volume, red blood cell mass and extracellular fluid space in man using radioactive I^{131}, $S^{35}O_4$, and Cr^{51}.* J Lab Clin Med 55:776, 1960.
25. SHIRES, GT, CUNNINGHAM, JN, AND BARKER, CRF: *Alterations in cellular membrane function during hemorrhagic shock in primates.* Ann Surg 176:288, 1972.
26. CUNNINGHAM, JN, SHIRES, GT, AND WAGNER, Y: *Cellular transport defects in hemorrhagic shock.* Surgery 70:215, 1971.
27. GILLON, J, ET AL: *A bioassay of treatment of hemorrhagic shock.* Arch Surg 93:537, 1966.
28. FULTON, RL: *The absorption of sodium and water by collagen during hemorrhagic shock.* Ann Surg 172:861, 1970.
29. GRAYSON, TL, LOHETE, JE, AND MOYER, CA: *Oxygen consumptions, concentrations of inorganic ions in urine, serum, and duodenal fluid, hematocrit, urinary excretion, pulse rates and blood pressure during duodenal depletion of sodium salts in normal and alcoholic man.* Ann Surg 158:840, 1963.
30. PAPPENHEIMER, JR AND SOTO-RIVERA, A: *Effective osmotic pressure of the plasma proteins and other quantities associated with the capillary circulation in the hind limbs of cats and dogs.* Am J Physiol 152:471, 1948.
31. BRIGHAM, KL, WOLVERTON, WC, AND BLAKE, HL: *Increased sheep lung vascular permeability caused by pseudomonas bacteremia.* J. Clin Invest 54:792, 1974.
32. ZARINS, CK, ET AL: *Lymph and pulmonary response to isobaric resuscitation in plasma oncotic pressure in baboons.* Circ Res 43:925, 1978.
33. PONTOPPIDAN, H, GEFFIN, B, AND LOWENSTEIN, E: *Acute respiratory failure in the adult.* N Eng J Med 287:690, 1972.
34. ROTHSCHILD, MA, ORATZ, M, AND SCHREIBER, SS: *Albumin metabolism.* Gastroenterology 64:324, 1973.
35. LEDGERWOOD, AM AND LUCAS, CE: *Postresuscitation hypertension, etiology, morbidity and treatment.* Arch Surg 108:531, 1974.
36. KOVALIK, SG, ET AL: *The cardiac effect of altered calcium homeostasis after albumin resuscitation.* J Trauma 21:275, 1981.
37. CORGAN, AG, ET AL: *The effect of crystalloid resuscitation in hemorrhagic shock on acid-base balance: A comparison between normal saline and Ringer's lactate solutions.* Surgery 69:874, 1971.

38. MESSMER, K, ET AL: *Oxygen transport and tissue oxygenation during hemodilution with dextran.* Adv Exp Med Biol 373:669, 1973.
39. REPLOGLE, RL, JUNDSLER, H, AND GROSS, RE: *Studies on the hemodynamic importance of blood viscosity.* J Thorac Cardiovasc Surg 50:658, 1965.
40. LAZROVE, S, ET AL: *Hemodynamic, blood volume and oxygen transport responses to albumin and hydroxyethyl starch infusions in critically ill postoperative patients.* Crit Care Med 8:302, 1980.
41. DAGHER, FJ, ET AL: *Blood volume measurement: A critical study. Prediction of normal values: Controlled measurement of sequential changes: Choice of a bedside method.* In: *Advances in Surgery,* C. E. Welch (ed), Chicago, Yearbook Medical Publishers, 1965.
42. CARRICO, CJ, CRENSHAW, CA, AND SHIRES, GT: *Effect of vasomotor drugs on the extracellular fluid volume during hemorrhagic shock.* Clin Res 10:288, 1962.

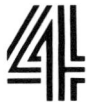

INTRAOPERATIVE FLUID THERAPY IN PEDIATRICS

Frederic A. Berry, M.D.

Deeply ingrained in the clinical folklore of medicine is the concept that newborns are totally salt intolerant. Evidence indicates, *au contraire,* that healthy term infants are capable of handling salt and water in a fashion similar to that of adults. The dogma of salt intolerance in this group of patients has led to many disasters and near-calamities as major deficits in plasma and extracellular volume were left untreated. Dr. F. A. (Fritz) Berry addresses this and other issues concerning controversies of fluid therapy in pediatric patients. Years ago it was unusual to start an intravenous line in the typical pediatric patient for surgery; now the reverse is true. Dr. Berry brings up many cogent points that are clinically relevant and pragmatic. One that caught my attention, and which was certainly ubiquitously true in the past, and may still be found here and there is the use of diuretics to increase urinary output during surgery. In fact, if there is a major deficit of plasma volume or extracellular fluid volume, diuretics, whether renal or osmotic, are the worst possible imposition on the patient, as they produce even more deficits in these volumes. Many times a cyclic disaster is produced. When urinary output reduces further, the cry of "oliguric renal shutdown" may be raised. This causes further reduction in the rate of administration of needed intravenous fluids. The correct and salubrious therapy is administration of sufficient fluid volume to make up for losses, however arcane they may be.

Burnell R. Brown, Jr.

The object of this chapter is to assist the clinician to evaluate the fluid and electrolyte status of the pediatric surgical patient, to manage intraoperative fluid therapy, and to provide postoperative follow-up. Fluid therapy should be continuous from patients' initial evaluation of until they are discharged from care. The spectrum of therapy varies from full resuscitation of the acutely ill patient to minimal fluid therapy in the child undergoing short, nontraumatic surgery. It is hoped that the material presented here will enable the clinician to manage the fluid continuum in a relatively simple and easy-to-remember fashion.

RENAL FUNCTION IN THE INFANT

In discussing any topic concerned with pediatrics, the enormous range of size and the range of maturation of the various organ systems are complicating factors. The most rapid change occurs at birth, with the transition of the fetus to the newborn. The neonatal period is usually defined as the first month of life. This is the period of the greatest changes in life: the transition from a physiologically dependent state to one in which the newborn and later the neonate must perform physiologic functions with support from the human environment. The transition process may be complicated by birth asphyxia, or prematurity, or both.[1] Since this chapter deals with fluid therapy, the transition of the kidney from a passive to an active organ is our major concern. However, individual organ maturation does not occur alone, but is dependent on successful transition of the body's other organ systems, such as the cardiopulmonary system and the central nervous system.

Renal maturation is of concern for those clinicians dealing with full-term and premature infants. Textbooks concerned with physiology of the newborn infant often report that variables of renal function, such as the glomerular filtration rate as determined by creatinine clearance, do not achieve adult values until 6 to 12 months of age.[2,3] But when one considers the functional abilities of the newborn and neonatal kidney, there is a different message. Normally, during the first 24 to 48 hours of life, there is a period when renal function undergoes a rapid transition from the passive fetal state to the active newborn state. All variables of renal function are very low at this point. However, in 4 to 5 days, even in the moderate sized premature infant, renal function rapidly improves. By one month of age, even though renal function variables are not those of an adult, they indicate that the infant's kidney is capable of withstanding severe challenges. Obviously, the cardiopulmonary and renal systems of the neonate must achieve a high degree of functional ability by 3 to 4 weeks of age, since it is not unusual for maintenance fluids in the premature infant to be in the range of 175 ml per kg per day, and for the full-term newborn to be 150 ml per kg per day. For the 70-kg man this represents approximately 10 liters per day. Regardless of what the normal adult values are for renal function, the numbers for performance are very impressive.

In summary, if renal maturation is judged by variables of renal function, such as the glomerular filtration rate, marked deficiency in renal function for the first several months of life would be indicated. However, when considered on a performance basis, that is, the ability to regulate the fluid volumes of the body, excrete various metabolites, and regulate electrolytes, the infant's kidney functions well after the initial transition phase.[4] In practical terms, when the transition is at its maximum in the first 24 hours of life, there is a reduced need for maintenance fluids and a decrease in the ability of the kidney to tolerate deficiencies or excesses of fluids. The therapeutic index is low. By four days of age there is marked improvement in renal function, and by a month of extrauterine life, the renal system is quite capable when considered on a performance basis.

PREOPERATIVE EVALUATION AND PREPARATION

The foundation for intraoperative fluid therapy is established by the preoperative evaluation and preparation of the patient. The healthy patient for elective surgery needs little, if anything, in the way of preoperative preparation. At the other end of the spectrum of evaluation and preparation is the patient who is desperately ill. Unless the patient is on the verge of a fatal hemorrhage requiring immediate definitive surgery, time must be taken to bring the patient rapidly into the best possible cardiopulmonary and fluid balance status. The anesthesiologist must be able to evaluate the fluid status of the patient and correct existing deficits. This requires a knowledge of (1) the content of the various fluid losses of the body, that is, upper gastrointestinal tract, lower gastrointestinal tract, traumatic edema, and so on; (2) what the extent of the losses are as judged by compensatory responses of the body to these losses; (3) fluid required to replace the deficit in both quantity and quality; and (4) the point at which the deficit has been adequately replaced, permitting the safe conduct of anesthesia.

The spectrum between the desperately ill child and the completely normal child for nontraumatic elective surgery includes a small group of children who require various diagnostic and therapeutic maneuvers to prepare them for surgery. Extensive diagnostic studies often require the patient to have prolonged periods without oral intake (NPO). This may lead to a subtle but important state of altered nutrition and fluid balance. Additional fluid deficits may occur when various diagnostic studies are performed involving the use of intravenous dyes that are osmotic diuretics, such as intravenous pyelograms (IVP), aortograms, and similar studies. The result of an osmotic diuretic may be the paradox of a dehydrated patient with a "good" urine output. Patients undergoing bowel surgery often have bowel preparation involving clear fluids and enemas. Because this may result in the loss of electrolytes, fluid, and nutrition, preoperative evaluation of the patient should specifically include these possibilities.

While the patient may be able to compensate for isolated challenges to fluid stability described above, when several of the factors are simultaneously operative, the effects become cumulative. In addition, the infant or child may be faced with the problem of fasting. The fasting period in healthy older children is usually of minor significance. In younger children and infants, however, fasting may lead to problems of dehydration and hypoglycemia. A trend toward shorter and more reasonable periods of being NPO has therefore developed in recent years. This is particularly important in infants, where the fluid loss per hour of being NPO is approximately double that in older children or adults. This latter group loses 4 percent of body weight after 24 hours of fasting, but the small infant will lose 10 percent. Hypoglycemia may occur secondary to long periods without oral intake, resulting in acidosis. Another reason for this approach is a humane one. It is very difficult for the infant, young child, and mother to cope with starvation and dehydration. One approach to the NPO period is:

Neonates	4 hours——milk	
	2 hours——clear fluids	
Infants	6 hours——milk	
	3 hours——clear fluids	
Children	4–6 hours——clear fluids	

It is clear that a number of factors may be operative in patients as they present for anesthesia and surgery. The body often is able to compensate partially or fully for these various challenges to fluid balance. However, the combination of several of these factors, together with the challenge of anesthesia and surgery, may overwhelm compensatory mechanisms, causing problems that recognition of the interplay of these factors and appropriate intraoperative fluid and electrolyte therapy might have forestalled.

Compensatory Mechanism for Fluid Loss

An elaborate system of compensatory mechanisms protects the body from the loss of fluids. Part of the preoperative preparation of the patient is recognizing when these compensatory mechanisms are in order. Activation of these compensatory systems generates various signs and symptoms that the clinician may recognize.[5]

Compensatory mechanisms for fluid loss are of two major kinds: temporary and definitive. Temporary mechanisms are activated to protect the circulating fluid volume, while definitive mechanisms replenish lost fluids and electrolytes. The temporary measures are those of translocation of fluids, release of antidiuretic hormone (ADH) to conserve water, and elaboration of endogenous vasopressors. The primary definitive mechanism to restore body fluid and electrolyte levels to normal is the renin-angiotensin-aldosterone (RAA) system. Major fluid losses by the body, as from the gastrointestinal tract or from trauma, are very high in sodium content. In fact, upper gastrointestinal tract losses and all losses of trauma can be considered full-strength losses and should be replaced with full-strength balanced salt solution, that is, full-strength saline, lactated Ringer's, or similar fluid. Glucose requirements will be covered below.

Temporary Compensatory Mechanisms

The rapid loss of fluid and electrolytes from the body may challenge the adequacy of the circulation to meet tissue perfusion needs. The process involving the translocation of extracellular fluid from the interstitial fluid volume into the plasma volume to help maintain a normal circulation is a temporary measure, and this fluid must be replenished. The signs of a loss of fluid from the interstitial space are a decrease in skin turgor, sunken fontanelles, and sunken eyeballs. Other temporary compensatory mechanisms involve the release of endogenous vasopressors and ADH. Most clinicians are well aware of the release of the catecholamines, epinephrine, and nonepinephrine, which lead to both peripheral vasoconstriction and beta effects on the myocardium. However, there are several other vasopressors which are also very important in temporary support of the circulation while definitive replacement therapy is being carried out. These are vasopressin, also known as ADH, and angiotensin II, which is part of the renin-angiotensin-aldosterone system.[6] Vasopressin has two effects on the body's compensatory system for fluid loss: (1) antidiuretic effect for the conservation of water and (2) vasoconstrictor effect. The role of vasopressin and angiotensin II is primarily that of vasoconstriction, resulting in an increase venous return in an attempt to maintain blood pressure.

Definitive Compensatory Mechanisms

The definitive compensatory mechanism for the replacement of lost body fluid is the RAA system, with an emergency backup by the ADH system for the retention of water. When there is a loss of sodium from the body there is an activation of the RAA system which ultimately leads to a release of aldosterone from the adrenal gland. Aldosterone circulates to the kidney, specifically to the distal tubule, where sodium and water are reabsorbed to a very high degree to replenish extracellular fluid volume. Signs of activation of this system are a decrease in urine sodium and a decrease in urine volume. If adequate sodium and water are given, this compensatory mechanism will be able to restore body fluid compartments to normal. However, the nature and degree of fluid loss often are not appreciated, and inappropriate fluid therapy, such as quarter strength saline, is used to replenish full strength losses. The continued loss of extracellular fluid and replacement by fluid low in sodium results in a sodium deficit. Since sodium normally determines the circulating blood volume, this deficit represents a volume challenge to the body. In the absence of adequate replacement sodium, the body turns to excess water being administered to restore the volume. The mechanism involves the release of ADH. This circulates to the distal tubule, where it acts to cause a reabsorption of free water, resulting in a progressive dilutional hyponatremia with the various sequelae including seizures, coma, and so forth. This is termed appropriate secretion of ADH and should not be confused with inappropriate secretion of ADH.

Summary of Preoperative Preparation

The clinician must evaluate the patient's fluid and electrolyte status preoperatively and, when indicated, provide adequate preoperative therapy before beginning anesthesia and surgery. The administration of anesthetics in the presence of hypovolemia with the activation of endogenous vasopressors may result in circulatory collapse. Adequate preparation of the patient includes close attention to urine output, which should be at the rate of one ml per kg per hour, as well as normal vital signs, tissue turgor, and fontanelles. In addition, electrolyte values should be returning to normal.

INTRAOPERATIVE FLUID THERAPY

Every patient for surgery does *not* need an IV. The indications for starting an IV include the condition of the patient, the type of surgery, and the need to administer drugs. If a patient has a short period of being NPO, and the surgery is short and nontraumatic, an IV may not be necessary—perhaps desirable but not mandatory. However, if the period of being NPO is prolonged, especially in the small infant, the problem of dehydration may be complicated by hypoglycemia. This may lead to postoperative depression, thereby prolonging the period without oral intake. A vicious cycle may ensue. If surgery is painful, the use of titrated intravenous narcotics is the most effective way to relieve discomfort. This need may justify the starting of an IV on this basis alone.

Intraoperative fluids can be divided into two major types: maintenance fluids and replacement fluids. Obviously, the body has an ever-present need for maintenance fluids to sustain normal fluid and electrolyte balance. Maintenance fluids are required for excretion of solutes, for water for the lungs and skin, and so forth. Some surgical procedures result in insignificant trauma to the body and subsequently no traumatic fluid loss. These procedures can be seen as maintenance-type procedures where maintenance-type fluids are quite satisfactory. Maintenance fluids are quarter strength saline or similar fluid. Other surgery involves varying degrees of trauma to the body and a loss of extracellular fluid, that is, plasma or interstitial fluid, or both. Therefore, for any surgery that may involve trauma and resulting loss of body fluids, balanced salt solution should be administered. The sodium content of these fluids is essentially the same as extracellular fluid.

The quandary of whether maintenance or replacement fluids should be given is simplified by two factors. The first is that the kidney has an enormous capability to excrete an overload of sodium, except for the first 24 hours of life. The second is that in maintenance-type surgery the period of fluid therapy is short, usually 1 to 2 hours, and relatively moderate amounts of sodium and fluid are administered. There is no danger of overloading the patient. For these reasons replacement fluids can be administered to all patients. In addition, the use of this type of fluid allows a degree of reserve in nontraumatic surgery, where postoperative problems such as vomiting may cause excessive loss of sodium, and maintenance fluids are not adequate to replace this loss. Severe derangements of fluids and electrolytes may occur, with disastrous results. It is therefore my practice to start balanced salt solution in all patients. All fluids should contain sodium. There is no place in pediatric fluid therapy for the use of plain glucose in water.

How much glucose to administer to pediatric patients is a persisting question. There are two potential problems. The first is that the pediatric patient has energy needs that must be met to avoid the onset of hypoglycemia. This may lead to temporary or long-term central nervous system problems, depending on the degree of hypoglycemia and the age of the patient. The second problem is hyperglycemia and the potential for hyperosmolar coma. This is more a theoretic problem than a practical one when glucose administered is in the range of 2½ to 5 percent. On the other hand, hyperalimentation fluids can easily cause hyperglycemia. Hyperglycemia may cause a diuresis, but clinical complications associated with this have not been a major problem. At this time the potential problems of hypoglycemia appear to exceed those of hyperglycemia and thus glucose should be administered to all patients. If more than one IV is running, only one IV needs the glucose. If hyperalimentation fluids are administered preoperatively, they should not be discontinued abruptly before surgery, since this may lead to a reactive hypoglycemia. There are two ways to prevent the problem: administration of 5 percent glucose with all fluids intraoperatively, or continuation of the hyperalimentation fluids at the preoperative rate. If fluid or blood volume deficits develop preoperatively or intraoperatively, they should be replaced with appropriate fluids. Hyperalimentation fluids should not be used to replace fluid or blood volume deficits.

Intraoperative fluid therapy has three goals: (1) to replace any deficits in maintenance fluids and to keep abreast of maintenance requirements; (2) to replace third space losses occurring because of tissue trauma; and (3) to replace blood loss with either blood or crystalloid, or a combination thereof, depending upon the clinical circumstances. Obviously, fluid therapy is a full spectrum, with some patients needing only minimal therapy, while others need maximum treatment. The following discussion offers guidelines for the administration of intraoperative fluids based on this spectrum. If the response to fluid therapy as reflected in vital signs, urine output, CVP, and so forth, indicates inadequate volume, more fluids are needed. If the response indicates that the patient's needs are being exceeded, fluids should be decreased. Fluid therapy is a dose-response relationship. The guidelines give initial dosages; response to therapy will determine subsequent doses.

The first hour of fluid therapy is concerned with the administration of a hydrating solution. For patients under 3 years of age, the amount given in the first hour is 25 ml per kg; for patients over 3 years, 15 ml per kg. This may seem like a large amount of fluid, but when the fact that most infants come to the operating room having been NPO for 4 to 12 hours is considered, these are reasonable volumes to restore this deficit. The average maintenance fluid need for children is 4 ml per kg per hour.[7] For young infants the figure is closer to 6 ml per kg per hour, and for older children (over 3 years) the amount is 2 ml per kg per hour. If surgery is brief and the child awakens rapidly, there is a good chance the IV will infiltrate. For this reason fluids should be administered fast enough to replace existing deficits before the IV is lost. This reduces the need to rush oral fluids postoperatively to insure that the child is hydrated.

Longer periods of surgery require fluids for the trauma of surgery plus the basic maintenance amounts. The trauma includes not only fluid that is lost in the sponges and tissues, but also blood loss. Blood loss replacement will be discussed below. The fluid that is translocated into the third space is extracellular fluid, with the same electrolyte value as plasma. Physically, the fluid is still within the confines of the body, and will appear on the scales as weight.[8] Functionally, however, it has been lost from the effective extracellular fluid volume and must be replaced. In mild trauma the loss is estimated at 2 ml per kg per hour, in moderate trauma it is 4 ml per kg per hour, and in severe trauma it is 6 ml per kg per hour. This fluid is given in addition to the basic maintenance fluid of 4 ml per kg per hour. The total fluid given for mild, moderate, or severe trauma is as follows:

Basic 4 ml/kg/hr + Mild Trauma 2 ml/kg/hr = 6 mg/kg/hr
Basic 4 ml/kg/hr + Moderate Trauma 4 ml/kg/hr = 8 ml/kg/hr
Basic 4 ml/kg/hr + Severe Trauma 6 ml/kg/hr = 10 ml/kg/hr.

This fluid is replaced with balanced salt solution. Keep in mind that these are guidelines. If urine output dwindles, more fluid is needed. If urine output is excessive, that is, more than 3 ml per kg per hour, less fluid is needed. The desired urine output during surgery is 1 to 2 ml per kg per hour. This is slightly higher than during the nonsurgical period, when it is usually ½ to 1 ml per kg per hour, but it makes the measurement of the urine volume more accurate.

The third goal of fluid therapy is to replace blood loss. Blood loss may be replaced with blood or with balanced salt solution, or with a combination of both. The condition of the patient and the type of surgery determine which approach to follow. Before surgery begins, there should be a discussion with the surgeon to determine anticipated blood loss. A value judgment is required to determine whether blood loss needs to be replaced immediately, or if it may be replaced with balanced salt solution. If the surgery is intracranial, cardiac, or on major blood vessels, the potential for rapid, relatively uncontrolled blood loss necessitates use of blood to replace blood loss as the bleeding occurs. When control of bleeding is not a problem, blood loss may be replaced with balanced salt solution up to about 20 percent of loss of blood volume. An example of this calculation is a 5-month-old infant weighing 5 kg on whom abdominal surgery will be performed. In infants and children 8 percent of body weight is blood volume. In adult males, 8 percent of body weight is blood volume and, in adult females, 7 percent is blood volume. In obese patients there is relatively less blood volume per body weight, and the figure drops to 7 percent and 6 percent of body weight for men and women respectively. In the example given, 5 kg $\times$ 8 percent equals 400 ml of blood volume. As a guideline, 20 percent of 400 ml equals 80 ml of possible allowable blood loss. The reduction in hematocrit should also be estimated. If the starting hematocrit is 36, then 20 percent of 36 equals 7. A hematocrit of 36 minus 7 results in a potential finishing hematocrit of 29. Assuming that appropriate replacement fluid is given to replace the blood loss, serial intraoperative hematocrits will help to reflect the amount of blood loss. A hematocrit of 28 to 30 is certainly an acceptable value in the postoperative period in patients who are otherwise healthy and are recovering from their surgery. The blood replacement formula is 3 to 4 ml balanced salt solution for every 1 ml blood loss. The reason for the extra fluid is that any sodium given will equilibrate itself between plasma volume and interstitial fluid, whereas the red cells stay with the blood volume.

The general condition of the infant is another factor that determines whether to replace blood loss with blood. If the child has been critically ill, blood loss greater than 5 percent of blood volume probably should be replaced with blood. Once more, this is a judgment decision, and these are guidelines.

Three factors in the transport of oxygen to cells are (1) hemoglobin, (2) cardiac output, and (3) ventilation. The delivery of oxygen to the cell depends upon all three factors. A drop in the hemoglobin is allowable within prescribed limits if the patient is able to increase cardiac output and if ventilation is adequate to insure an oxygen saturation of 90 to 95 percent. However, if heart disease or respiratory disease is present, affecting the ability to compensate for a drop in hemoglobin, blood loss must be replaced with blood to insure adequate oxygen delivery to tissues.

Patient Monitoring

The patient must be monitored. The basic monitors are chest stethoscope, blood pressure, electrocardiogram (ECG), and temperature. If a potential blood loss of 15 to 20 percent of blood volume is anticipated, consideration should be given to use of various invasive monitors. Urine output monitoring should be seriously considered. Using a direct arterial line in patients whose blood loss may approach 20 percent of blood volume offers the safety and simplicity of a constant readout and the availability of blood for measurement of blood gases and other purposes. The degree of blood loss and basic condition of the patient may indicate a need for additional monitors such as a CVP or a Swan-Ganz catheter. Monitoring techniques other than the basic ones are dictated by the experience of the clinician, the condition of the patient, and the nature of the surgery. The recent introduction of automatic time-cycled blood pressure devices with a digital readout greatly enhances the clinician's ability to rapidly determine changes in vital signs.

Intraoperative Hypotension

If hypotension develops, the clinician must have in mind an automatic checklist to run through to determine the reason for the hypotension. It should be noted that there are occasions when it appears that a drop in blood pressure is a mechanical problem associated with the monitor rather than with the patient. Such a drop in pressure should always be assumed to be a problem with the patient rather than with the monitor. A complete check must be made of the patient's condition and the anesthetic system. If nothing is found, and the patient's condition is at variance with what is suggested by the blood pressure, it may be assumed that there is a problem with the monitor. This sequence should not occur in reverse because valuable time may be lost while it is discovered that the monitor is accurate and the patient is in serious difficulty.

The basic reasons for hypotension are (1) interference with oxygenation, (2) myocardial compromise, and (3) inadequate circulating blood volume. There is relatively little innovative thinking in an acute emergency. The clinician must therefore have, in addition to a checklist of possible causes of the hypotension, a set of therapeutic maneuvers to correct the problem temporarily and then definitively. If the onset of hypotension is sudden, the anesthetic should be turned off immediately and ventilation with oxygen insured. At the same time, the circulating blood volume should be augmented by turning up the IV, and if blood is not being given, its use strongly considered. If the pressure has dropped to alarmingly low levels, the use of inotropic and chronotropic agents should be considered to temporarily augment the circulation while definitive measures are being completed. The slow onset of hypotension provides the clinician more time to better determine the cause of the difficulty. Once more, a checklist will facilitate rapid systematic evaluation of the problem. The list again begins with a basic check of the anesthetic system to determine (1) that adequate oxygen is being supplied, (2) the concentration of anesthetics being administered, and (3) the adequacy of ventilation. Fluids should be increased. If the surgery involves blood loss, a check and recalculation should be made of the degree of such blood loss. It is very difficult to measure and estimate blood loss in small children, in spite of all the contrivances available to assist a determination. If in doubt, blood should be administered. Calcium is an excellent cardiotonic drug, and consideration should be given to administering a dose of approximately 50 to 100 mg per kg over 10 minutes.[9] Slowly dropping blood pressure is usually due to inadequate fluid replacement.

Summary of Intraoperative Fluid Therapy

Intraoperative fluids require a plan with respect to the preoperative condition of the patient and the intraoperative needs. The amount of fluids recommended are suggested as guidelines. It is the response of the patient to the fluid amounts that determine any changes in the amount of IV fluid given. There is no set of magical numbers which can be determined before surgery and continued throughout the surgical period without regard to the response of the patient.

THE POSTOPERATIVE PERIOD

There is a misconception among some clinicians that the end of surgery is accompanied by an end to the loss of fluid by damaged tissue. Unfortunately, this is not true. Trauma to tissue results in interruption of normal cellular integrity, leading to translocation of fluid into the third space. Until the cell restores this integrity, the loss of fluid continues. If the surgery is minor, compensation for the loss of tissue fluid into the third space is accomplished by the normal compensatory mechanisms described above. However, the ability of the compensatory system to effectively compensate for the loss of tissue fluid varies inversely with the degree of trauma. Unfortunately, most clinicians feel that tissue trauma has ceased in the postoperative period and therefore convert the replacement fluid, balanced salt solution, to maintenance fluids such as quarter strength saline. The degree of trauma and the ability of the patient to compensate will determine whether these fluids are adequate or inadequate. The use of the correct fluid greatly increases the chance of physiologic restitution of the patient's losses. If inadequate fluids and electrolytes are given, usually the first reaction is a drop in urine volume or in serum sodium. A drop in urine volume can be caused by any of three mechanisms: (1) a problem with myocardial function, (2) a problem of renal function, and (3) inadequate fluid volume and content. In healthy patients with no previous heart disease, it is highly unlikely that the problem lies within the cardiovascular system. The same can be said of the kidneys. The most frequent cause of a decrease in urine output in the postoperative period is inadequate fluid volume and inadequate fluid content.[10] The problem is that traumatized tissue continues to lose fluid that contains sodium in the same amount as serum levels, and the fluid is often replaced with quarter strength saline. There remains a small but unfortunately determined group of clinicians who diagnose this problem as an "inborn error of Lasix or Mannitol metabolism." In the postoperative period when urine output drops, their first therapy option is to treat symptomatically the decrease in urine by the administration of a diuretic. Any patient with a decrease in urine output following surgery needs to have a bolus of balanced salt solution administered. The dose is 10 ml per kg per hour. Too often we overlook the fact that the kidney regulates fluids and electrolytes; it does not create them.

In recognition of the fact that ideal fluid management of the patient as judged by our surgical and pediatric colleagues is probably an unobtainable goal, achievable clinical objectives need to be set. The choice is whether the patient is to receive less than ideal management or more than than ideal management. This is a choice not unlike the length of a suture being too long or too short. Are patients better served by giving too little fluid, that is, keeping them dry, or by small excesses of fluid to insure a normal circulation and extra urine? The pharmacologic concept of the therapeutic index of fluids should be considered. On the low side there is a minimal tolerance level, the amount of fluid the body needs as an absolute minimum to maintain its normal functions. On the high side there is a maximal tolerance level; above this there are problems with circulatory overload. In the first days of life the therapeutic range index is rather narrow; the therapeutic index being approximately 3 to 1, maximal to minimal tolerance. However, by 1 month of age, the maximal to minimal tolerance ratio is about 10 to 1. Maintenance fluid estimates are usually the minimal tolerance plus about 10 percent. For normal patients with no unexpected difficulties, this may be quite sufficient. However, this type of system has no reserve for possible complications such as nausea and vomiting, intestinal obstruction, occult bleeding, or continued extracellular fluid loss from trauma. Therefore, the philosophy of fluid balance advocated here is to stay on the generous side of the ideal amount, rather than on the minimal side of the ideal amount. The therapeutic objective is to give fluids and electrolytes adequate to allow the patient to correct ongoing losses, and allow a reserve for unexpected and unrecognized problems. Any excess can be excreted easily by the kidneys. The more extensive the trauma, the more important becomes attention to detail and results. This is particularly true now in severely traumatized patients who are a challenge not only in the operating room but, also in the recovery period in the surgical intensive care unit. Currently, there is considerable interest in the problem of the patient with developing renal failure and whether this is oliguric renal failure or nonoliguric renal failure.[10] Evidence is rapidly mounting that nonoliguric renal failure offers a better chance for patients' survival and quality of life. The clinical management of this most difficult problem requires the use of extensive invasive monitoring to determine the status of the myocardium, the fluid volume, and the vascular bed. These patients challenge the ingenuity and skill of the anesthesiologist.

SUMMARY

The practice of anesthesia embodies the concept of a dose-response curve. A dose of barbiturate is given, the response of the patient is judged, and the situation is then re-evaluated. End points are rather clear. If the patient is asleep, the dose is adequate; if the patient is not asleep, more is given. The same sort of dose-response relationships are also observed with narcotics, muscle relaxants, and similar medications. It is helpful to think of fluid and electrolytes in terms of a dose-response relationship. This will increase the clinician's appreciation of this very dynamic situation and lead to a better understanding of the process and better care of our patients.

REFERENCES

1. GREGORY, GA: *Resuscitation of the newborn.* Anesthesiology 43:225, 1975.
2. FANAROFF, AA AND KLAUS, MH: *Care of the High-Risk Neonate.* WB Saunders, Philadelphia, 1979, p 112.
3. BENNETT, EJ AND PAYNE, JP: *Fluids For Anesthesia and Surgery in the Newborn and the Infant.* Charles C Thomas, Springfield, Illinois, 1975
4. ROSS, B, COWETT, RM, AND OH, W: *Renal functions of low birth weight infants during the first two months of life.* Pediatr Res 11:1162, 1972
5. BEVAN, DR: *Renal Function in Anesthesia and Surgery.* Academic Press, London, 1979
6. MILLER, ED, ET AL: *Converting-enzyme activity and pressor responses to angiotensin I and II in the rat awake and during anesthesia.* Anesthesiology 50:88, 1979
7. FURMAN, EB, ET AL: *Specific therapy in water, electrolyte and blood-volume replacement during pediatric surgery.* Anesthesiology 42:187, 1975
8. SCHWARTZ, SI, ET AL: *Principles of Surgery.* McGraw-Hill, New York, 1969, p 31.
9. GREGORY, GA: *Newborn and Neonatal Emergency Anesthetics.* American Society of Anesthesiologists. 31st Annual Refresher Course Lectures, 1980
10. SHIN, B, ET AL: *Postoperative renal failure in trauma patients.* Anesthesiology 51:218, 1979

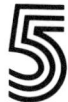

ROLE OF COLLOID OSMOTIC PRESSURE IN SHOCK RESUSCITATION*

Robert E. Drake, Ph.D., and
Joseph C. Gabel, M.D.

An ongoing debate, and one that frequently produces more heat than light, concerns the requirement for colloid solutions to prevent leakage of fluids into the lung. Several years ago the entity of post-traumatic wet lung (Danang lung) prompted many physicians to mix significant amounts of colloid solution (e.g., albumin) with crystalloid during resuscitation. With the expense and lack of availability of albumin, the need to use this preparation presents an extremely cogent clinical problem. Drs. Drake and Gabel, individuals who have been interested in permeability alterations of the lung, give a detailed explanation of the theory behind this problem in the following chapter. They indicate that a variety of factors are involved, and that the issue is—as might be expected—extremely complex. Without changes in permeability, almost regardless of plasma oncotic pressure, there will be little in the way of leakage into the alveoli. Their advice is to stay out of trouble, and to prevent pulmonary edema. Obviously this is not always possible. An important point is that once permeability changes have occurred, protein can extravasate extravascularly as well as water. This can compound the issue by taking with it water into the alveoli. Thus, it may be that once the critical changes observed by the authors have occurred, it may be too late for intravenous infusion of albumin or purified plasma fraction to be of any value. In fact, under the circumstances it may be harmful. However, this is a debatable issue that we will see recurring in the literature in years to come.

Burnell R. Brown, Jr.

---

*Much of this material was presented as an American Society of Anesthesiologists Annual Refresher Course Lecture in October 1981.

The means by which pressure and permeability changes affect transcapillary fluid exchange must be appreciated before an appropriate physiologic approach to therapy can be applied in shock. The changes in lung fluid exchange characteristics in shock will be discussed as being representative of the changes occurring in other vascular beds because the effects of such changes are clinically of paramount import. Pulmonary edema results from the inability of the pulmonary lymph system to remove fluid as rapidly as it is filtered through the vascular membranes. It is generally believed that this relative lymphatic insufficiency is caused by a higher than normal microvascular filtration rate, rather than an insufficient lymphatic system. Accordingly, most investigators have confined their efforts to studying the mechanisms of fluid filtration.

The rate at which fluid is filtered from the capillaries into the tissues is governed by the Starling equation:[1]

$$Jv = Kf[Pc - Pt - \sigma(\pi c - \pi t)]$$

where Kf = the capillary filtration coefficient, Pc = the capillary hydrostatic pressure, Pt = the tissue fluid hydrostatic pressure, σ = the capillary membrane reflection coefficient to proteins, πc = plasma oncotic pressure (colloid osmotic pressure), and πt = tissue fluid oncotic pressure (tissue colloid osmotic pressure). The Starling equation is simply another flow = pressure/resistance equation; pressure is the term in brackets, and Kf is the reciprocal of the resistance of the capillary membrane to fluid flow.

The pressure term of the Starling equation is composed of two parts: (1) the difference in hydrostatic pressure across the capillary membrane (Pc − Pt) and (2) the difference in oncotic pressure $[\sigma(\pi c - \pi t)]$. It is this separation of terms in the equation that has led to the "oncometer" concept of microvascular fluid exchange. According to this concept, hydrostatic pressure tends to push fluid into the tissues and the plasma oncotic pressure tends to cause reabsorption of this fluid. Thus, pressure edema can result only when Pc exceeds πc and pushes excessive amounts of fluid into the tissues.

The oncometer concept was first demonstrated in the lung by Guyton and Lindsey in 1959.[2] They increased the left atrial pressure in dogs and found that edema occurred only when the left atrial pressure exceeded πc. In animals in which they lowered πc by plasmaphoresis, the critical left atrial pressure was less. Although Guyton and Lindsey did not consider the importance of the other pressure terms in the

Starling equation, they did clearly demonstrate the importance of the oncotic effect on lung fluid balance. It is the oncometer concept that has led to a common clinical test for increased permeability. If a patient has pulmonary edema and an elevated left atrial pressure, the edema is believed to be hydrostatic; edema in a patient with low left atrial pressure is believed to indicate increased permeability.

Such a simplistic approach ignores basic science. It is not acceptable, in an already pathologic state, to assume that if one determinant of capillary pressure (left atrial pressure) is normal, then the cause of the pulmonary edema is increased permeability. Research in transcapillary fluid exchange has not focused on the development of clinically significant edema. In fact almost all research in lung fluid exchange, laboratory and clinical alike, has either been performed in normal nonedematous lungs or after the fact under grossly edematous conditions. An understanding of the terms of the Starling equation and how they are measured in the laboratory must form the real basis for evaluating the commonly accepted vascular changes in shock. Without a knowledge of the normal state (and a reproducible method of definition), the pathophysiology involved cannot be delineated.

THE CAPILLARY FILTRATION COEFFICIENT

Kf is a measure of the ease with which capillary filtrate moves through the capillary membrane. It is numerically equal to the filtration rate (milliliters per minute) for a unit pressure difference (millimeters of mercury) across the capillary membrane. It is usually expressed on a per unit weight basis (100 grams) and thus represents the sum of the filtration coefficients for all the capillaries in a unit of organ weight.

The first attempted measurement of Kf was made by Guyton and Lindsey.[2] They estimated the Kf to be 0.07 ml per minute per mmHg per 100 g. As was stated above, Guyton and Lindsey did not consider the changes in Pt, πt, and lymph flow rate ($\dot{Q}_L$) flow rate which occur in edema. Thus they may have underestimated Kf.

In an effort to circumvent the problem of these changes, later investigators used the change in weight of isolated lungs to estimate Kf. Since the weight could be measured continuously, it was possible to estimate Jv very soon after a change in Pc—possibly before changes in Pt, πt, or $\dot{Q}_L$ could occur. Kfs obtained by this method are generally larger than Guyton and Lindsey's; however, this could be due to changes in blood volume which affect the weight measurement. Also, isolated lungs are quite possibly affected by the isolation procedure.

(Morris reported threefold larger Kfs in isolated compared with non-isolated lungs.[3])

Aware of the problems with isolated lung preparations, Staub introduced a model in 1970[4] in which lymph could be collected from the lungs of unanesthetized, untraumatized sheep. Later, Erdmann and associates[5] used the sheep model to estimate Kf. They took the approach of measuring or estimating all the other terms in the Starling equation, and solving for Kf. They reasoned that because capillary filtrate is removed by the lymph system, the capillary filtration rate (Jv) would be equal to $\dot{Q}_L$ and the lymph oncotic pressure would equal πt. They calculated Pc from the pulmonary arterial and left atrial pressures, calculated πc from the plasma protein concentration, and assumed Pt to equal 0 and σ to equal 1.

Almost all studies have indicated that Pt is negative (not 0), and the assumption that σ was equal to 1 is probably incorrect, as they found the lymph (representing tissue fluid) to be rich in protein. If Erdmann had used a Pt of less than 0 and a σ of less than 1, his estimate of Kf would have been markedly different.

We have developed a preparation which allows us to avoid some of the trauma associated with the isolated lung preparation.[6] With this preparation, we can continuously monitor the intact lower left lobe weight of anesthetized open-chested dogs. Lobar arterial and venous pressures are controlled by electromechanical feedback systems. In order to estimate Kf, we increase Pc in steps. Once Pc exceeds a critical level, the lung weight begins to increase at a constant rate. We have been able to verify that at the time of our measurements, Kf, Pt, πt, and $\dot{Q}_L$ are not changing (as most certainly occurred in the experiments of Guyton and Lindsey). From the relationship between the rate of the weight gain and Pc, we have estimated Kf to be 0.10 ml per minute per mmHg per 100 g.

The importance of the actual value of Kf depends on the lymph flow rate. For example, the lymph flow rate may increase by a factor of 10 or more in edematous states, to a value in excess of 0.5 ml per minute per 100 g. The filtration coefficient determines how much pressure must exist across the capillary membrane to result in a fluid flux of 0.5 ml per minute ($\dot{Q}_L$/Kf). If Kf = 0.1, a pressure difference of only 5 mmHg would be required. If, however, Kf = 0.007, as estimated by Erdmann, the pressure drop across the membrane would have to be in excess of 70 mmHg.

The pressure drop across the capillary membrane required to cause a filtration rate equal to the maximum lymph flow rate is a "safety factor" against edema. If the Kf is more than 0.10 ml per minute per mmHg per 100 g, the safety factor is less than 5 mmHg, and is negligible compared with the capillary pressure required to cause edema. If Kf is less than 0.10, the lymph flow safety factor could play a substantial role in the ability of the lung to resist edema.

Capillary filtration is generally believed to occur in pores or slits between capillary endothelial cells. Thus, the Kf should depend upon the number and size of the pores. Owing to the relationship of the radius and the hydraulic conductivity of a pore, Kf should depend upon the fourth power of the pore radius. A change in microvascular permeability, manifested by a small increase in pore radius, should cause a very large increase in Kf. Thus Kf is one of the two terms in the Starling equation which is directly affected by changes in permeability (the other term is σ).[7]

TISSUE FLUID ONCOTIC PRESSURE

πt is another important safety factor against edema; the tissue fluid oncotic pressure is dependent upon a concentration of various protein factions in the fluids outside the capillary membrane. There are two ways protein molecules move from the plasma to tissue fluids: convection and diffusion.

If the pores of the membrane are larger than protein molecules, the protein will slowly diffuse into the tissue spaces and the tissue concentration will increase. If there is no net fluid filtration into the tissues, tissue concentration will eventually equal the plasma concentration. The rate at which protein diffuses into the tissues is equal to a diffusion coefficient, commonly called the permeability surface area product (PS), times the difference between the plasma and tissue (lymph) concentrations.

In a normal lung, fluid does filter across the capillary membrane. This fluid is removed by the lymphatic system, resulting in the continuous dilution of tissue proteins with a capillary filtrate. The removal of tissue protein by the lymph vessels prevents the tissue concentration from rising to equal the plasma concentration. Although the capillary filtrate dilutes tissue proteins, it also carries some protein into the tissues, because protein is dissolved in the filtrate. The total rate of protein transport through the capillary membrane is the sum of diffusion and convective transport. In general, when the capillary filtration rate increases, the tissue fluid protein concentration is decreased.

The decrease in tissue concentration was first observed by Drinker and Field.[8] They found that when they increased the left atrial pressure in dogs, the right lymph duct flow rate increased and the lymph protein concentration decreased. The absolute value of the minimum tissue concentration for protein is not known. In anesthetized, open-chested dogs, tissue concentration can be reduced to less than 50 percent of the plasma concentration by increasing the pulmonary capillary pressure. In anesthetized sheep, the tissue concentration may be reduced even further after several days of increased left atrial pressure.

The decrease in tissue concentration as the filtration rate across the capillary membrane increases causes πt to decrease. From the Starling equation this decrease in the πt tends to reduce the rate of fluid movement to a degree related to the effectiveness of the capillary membrane as a barrier to the free passage of protein. Thus the change in πt with increased Jv represents another safety factor against edema.

TISSUE FLUID HYDROSTATIC PRESSURE

Pt is the most controversial and difficult to measure of the pressures which affect microvascular filtration. Pt differs from the total tissue pressure because it does not include the pressure exerted by tissue fibers. Meyer, Meyer, and Guyton[9] made the first attempt to measure Pt. They implanted small porous plastic capsules in the lung tissue of dogs and allowed the wounds to heal. They then measured the pressure inside the hollow capsules as an estimate of Pt. The principle of the tissue capsules is that fluid pressure can equilibrate through the pores, but tissue fibers cannot grow into the center of the capsule for several months. Thus, at the center of the capsule, there is a space filled with fluid, the pressure of which can be measured. Meyer's group found that the Pt averaged -7 mmHg. They also showed that Pt rose to approximately 2 to 3 mmHg when they elevated left atrial pressure. Pt has also been estimated from the pressure of fluid in obstructed alveoli and in isolated dog lungs. These studies indicate that Pt is negative, but becomes 0 or positive as edema develops. Pt may reach a plateau as edema formation occurs. The increase in Pt which occurs as tissue fluid collects in the lung tends to reduce the rate of capillary filtration. Accordingly, this change in Pt is another safety factor against edema.

PULMONARY CAPILLARY PRESSURE

Pc, defined as the average hydrostatic pressure in the small pulmonary vessels in which filtration occurs, is not readily measurable; it is frequently estimated both experimentally and clinically by the equation:

$$Pc = Pv + \gamma(Pa - Pv)$$

where: γ is the ratio of the resistance downstream from the exchange vessels to total pulmonary vascular resistance, and Pa and Pv are pulmonary arterial and venous pressures respectively.

Early attempts at measuring Pc consisted of wedging small catheters into pulmonary arteries and measuring the pressure. Unfortunately, the wedged catheters blocked blood flow through the vascular bed in which they were located. Thus, the pressure actually measured was not the capillary pressure but the pressure in the venous system.

Gaar and associates[10] estimated Pc in isolated dog lungs. They perfused the lung and adjusted the venous pressure to obtain an isogravimetric state. They then lowered Pa and increased Pv to obtain another isogravimetric state, reasoning that Pc should be the same for each isogravimetric state. Therefore, as they repeated the procedure, Pa and Pv each approached Pc. They found that γ equals 0.44. We estimated γ in intact dog lungs with a similar technique to Garr's and obtained a value of 0.5.[11] Micropuncture studies of surface capillaries in isolated dog lungs and estimates of Pc from fluid-filled alveoli have also generally supported Garr's data.

A large fraction of the total pulmonary vascular pressure drop may be in the capillaries themselves. Furthermore, filtration may occur throughout the entire length of the capillaries as well as in the arterioles and venules. Therefore, the best estimate of Pc must be one which is an average of the pressures along the capillary. By using a technique which depended upon the filtration rate through the capillary membrane, Gaar's results should be a functional estimate of Pc.

Brody and Stemmler[12] first introduced a low viscosity bolus technique for estimating the resistance distribution in isolated lungs. Although this technique does not allow for the determination of the functional Pc, it has been used to estimate the change in the distribution of resistance caused by various factors.

Many investigators have used Gaar's estimate of the distribution of resistance to calculate Pc in various preparations. This equation may yield reasonable estimates of Pc under normal circumstances; however, various drugs and pathologic states may alter this ratio and could lead to a large error in the estimate of Pc.

THE REFLECTION COEFFICIENT

The reflection coefficient, σ, of the capillary membrane is different for different sized pores. A more correct expression for the osmotic term of the Starling equation would be the sum of all the oncotic pressures exerted by each protein fraction times the σ for that fraction. In the absence of quantitative data for the individual reflection coefficients, they have usually been combined into one term.

With the recent surge of interest in pulmonary lymph have come some techniques for estimating both σ and pore size (PS) for individual protein fractions. Two different categories of techniques have been used. Some investigators have developed mathematical models and used computers to determine what values of σ and PS would cause the models to best fit experimental data. Other investigators have applied various equations for protein transport to the lymph data to estimate σ and PS. Taylor, Granger, and Brace[13] have analyzed the lymph data from several different tissues. They assumed that the lymph flow rate was equal to the membrane filtration rate, and that the tissue concentration was equal to the lymph protein concentration. By analyzing the data at different lymph flow rates, they were able to estimate both σ and PS. This technique yielded plausible results for the data from several tissues and isolated dog lungs, but did not obtain meaningful results for sheep lung lymph data. For the isolated dog lung data, they found σ equals 0.73.

LYMPH FLOW

Drinker and Field[8] were the first to collect pulmonary lymph. Although they were not able to collect pure lung lymph, they demonstrated that pulmonary lymph flow increased when left atrial pressure was increased. Normand and associates[14] developed a technique for collecting lymph from the large caudal mediastinal lymph node in sheep. Most of the lung lymph passes through this node along with some nonpulmonary lymph. Staub later developed a technique to eliminate most of the nonpulmonary lymph in the sheep. Recently there have been several preparations developed to collect pulmonary lymph from dog lungs. Experiments with most of these preparations show that when left atrial pressure is increased, the lymph flow rate increases and the lymph protein concentration decreases. Several interesting and as yet unexplained results have come from recent lymph studies in dogs. As capillary pressures increase, lung lymph flow rate increases; however, when Pc exceeds critical level, the lymph flow rate reaches a plateau. Parker and associates[15] have noted a similar phenomenon in a study in which they infused lactated Ringer's solution into dogs and measured $\dot{Q}_L$. He has also shown that $\dot{Q}_L$ may decrease to below its maximum value even though the lung is grossly edematous. Presumably, this relative failure of the lymphatic system may result from the accumulation of fluid away from the terminal vessels.

THE TOTAL EDEMA SAFETY FACTOR

The intrinsic resistivity of the lung to edema formation has been called the pulmonary "safety factor." The total safety factor against edema is the sum of the lung's ability to alter tissue pressure (Pt), tissue fluid oncotic pressure (πt), and lymph flow rate ($\dot{Q}_L$). Although the magnitude of the individual factors are difficult to determine, the total safety factor can be determined by increasing the Pc to a lung and noting the lowest pressure at which edema begins to form. The total safety factor is the difference between this critical capillary pressure and the normal capillary pressure. We have performed this experiment and found that the critical pressure (Pc,critical) is a function of πc (Fig. 1). This result indicates that the magnitudes of the individual safety factors are set by the plasma oncotic pressure.

The fact that Pc,critical is a function of πc emphasizes the oncometer concept of pulmonary microvascular fluid exchange. The plasma oncotic pressure resists the movement of fluid into the tissues caused by elevated capillary hydrostatic pressure. Figure 1 shows that the greater the plasma oncotic pressure, the greater is the ability of the lung to resist edema formation.

The full oncotic pressure of protein can be exerted across the capillary membrane only if the protein molecules cannot penetrate the pores of the membrane. The presence of protein in tissue fluid indicates that the pulmonary microvascular membrane is not completely impermeable to protein. This effect is accounted for in the Starling equation by σ. There is a different σ for each protein fraction, the value of σ depending upon the relative size of the protein and the membrane pores. The larger the protein molecule relative to the membrane pores, the larger σ. σ for albumin has been estimated to be approximately

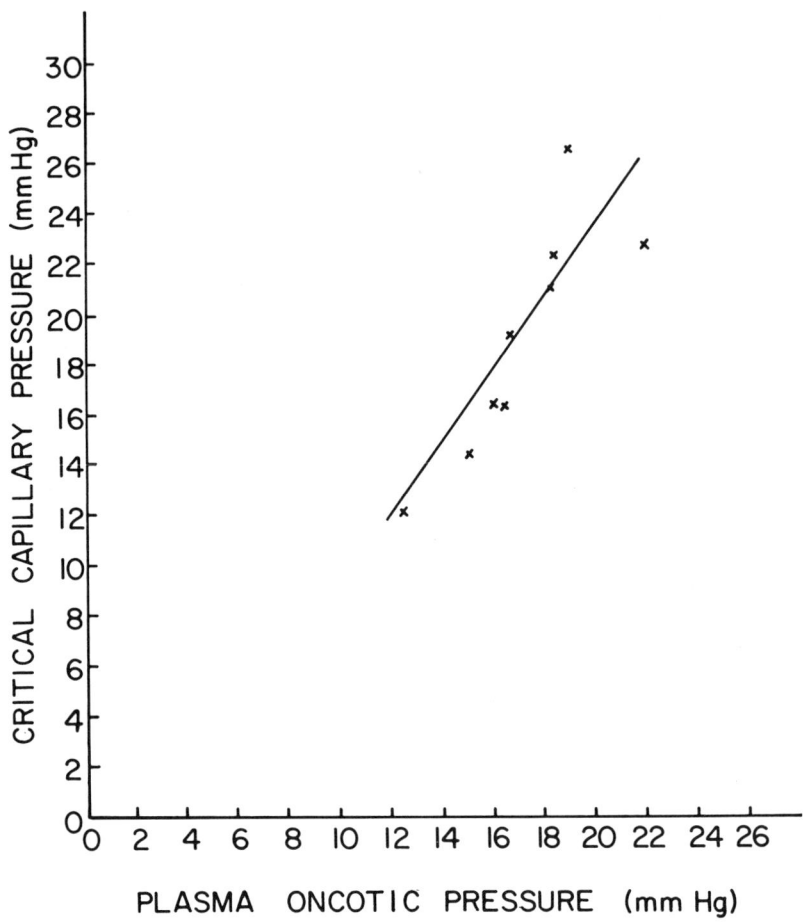

Figure 1. The relationship between the critical capillary pressure (Pc,critical) and the plasma oncotic pressure (πc) for each of nine experiments.

0.50 for dog lungs.[16] σ is approximately 0.9 to 1.0 for much larger protein molecules.

EFFECT OF INCREASED PERMEABILITY

σ for all protein molecules may be reduced by the administration of certain toxic agents. One such agent, alloxan, has been shown to cause large pores to occur in the capillary membrane. Theoretically, alloxan should thus cause a reduction in the effective oncotic pressure across the capillary membrane. This should reduce Pc,critical accordingly. Figure 2 shows Pc,critical versus πc for six dogs after the intravenous administration of 75 mg per kg of alloxan. In each experiment, Pc,critical was less than control, and in some lungs, Pc,critical was less than the capillary pressure (before we elevated Pc) so that spontaneous edema formation occurred.

It is clear from experiments such as those of Figure 2 that the plasma oncotic pressure has little effect on resisting edema formation when σ is greatly reduced (i.e., permeability is increased). There is

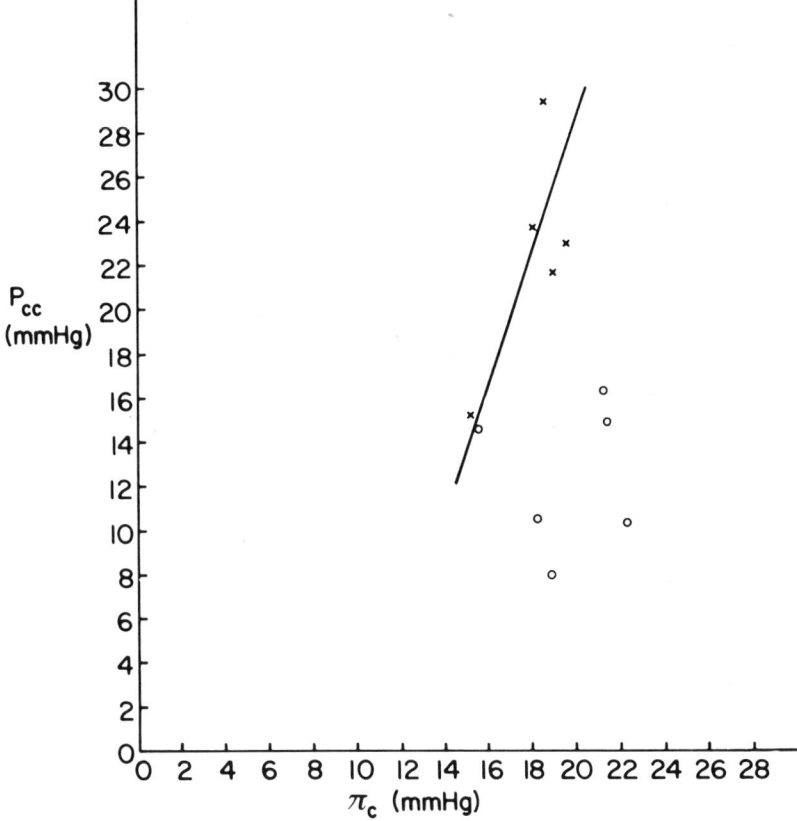

Figure 2. Critical capillary pressure (Pcc) vs. plasma oncotic pressure for 6 days after 75 mg per kg of alloxan (circles). Data for control dogs (xs) were consistent with Figure 1.

little experimental evidence that this degree of membrane damage occurs in sepsis. Figure 3 shows Pc,critical versus πc for experiments in which we gave dogs 4 mg per kg of E. coli endotoxin. The endotoxin did not reduce Pc,critical. Thus the plasma oncotic pressure was just as effective in resisting edema formation as it was in control animals. We obtained similar results during infusions of 4 mg per kg per minute of histamine phosphate (Fig. 4).

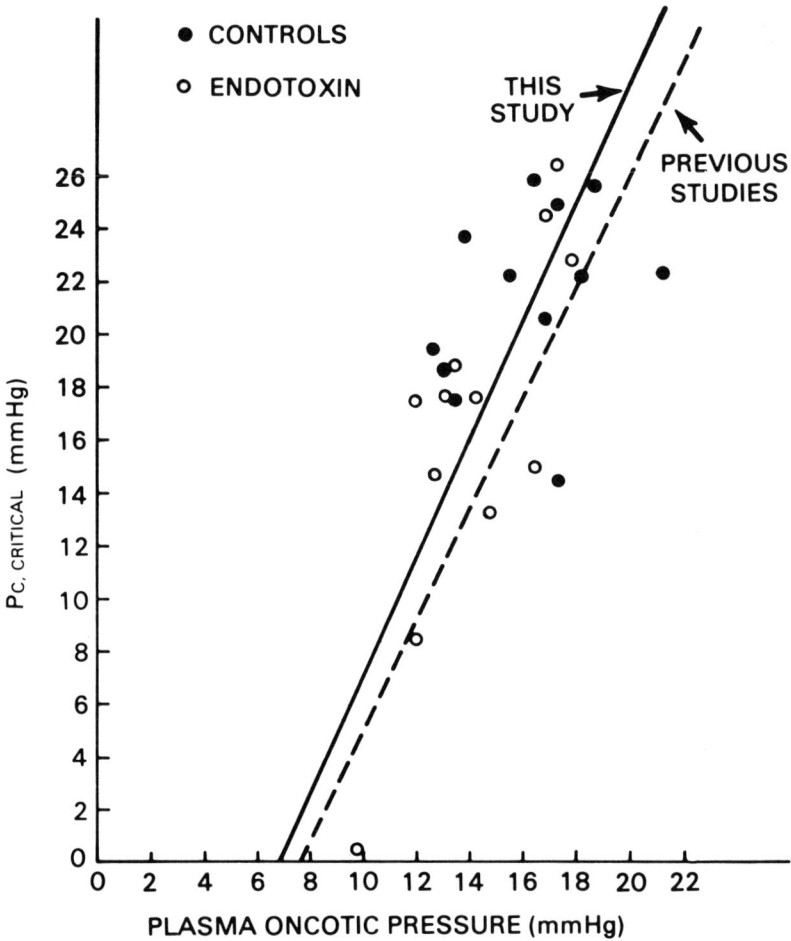

Figure 3. Pc,critical versus πc for control dogs and dogs given 4 mg per kg of E. coli endotoxin. The solid line is the least squares "best fit" line to the control experiments; the dashed line is the best fit line to the data from several previous studies.[6,7]

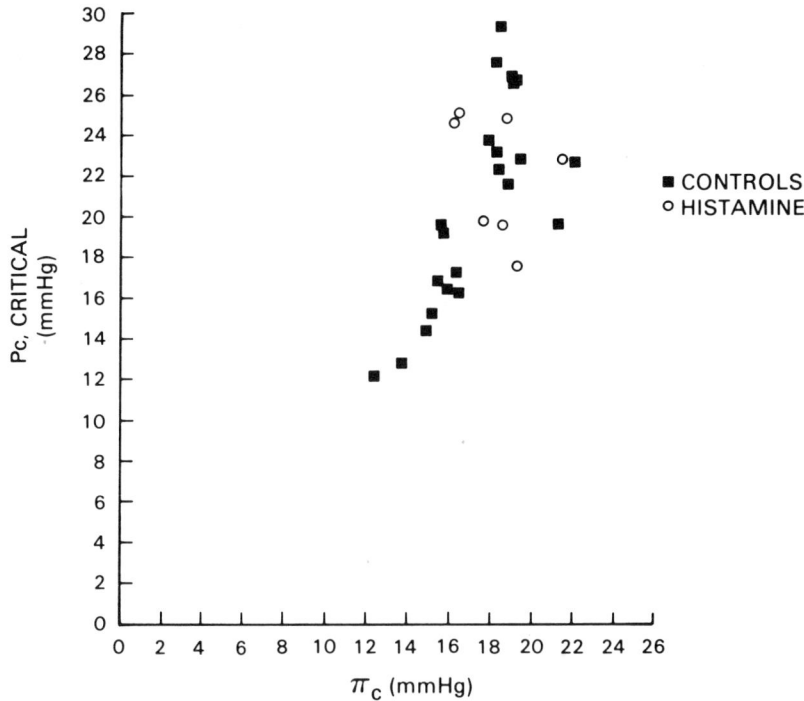

Figure 4. Pc,critical versus πc data for dogs during an infusion of 4 mg per kg per min of histamine phosphate. Also shown are Pc,critical vs. πc for control experiments.

OTHER PERMEABILITY STUDIES

In 1974, Brigham and associates[17] used the sheep lung preparation of Staub to detect increased permeability caused by pseudomonas bacteremia. They increased the left atrial pressure in seven sheep and found that lymph flow increased and lymph protein concentration decreased. They then decreased the left atrial pressure and infused pseudomonas bacteria intravenously. After pseudomonas, the lymph flow increased more and the lymph protein concentration decreased less than it had at increased left atrial pressure. They concluded that the pseudonomas had caused the permeability to increase. Following the initial pseudomonas study, this technique has been used to detect possible changes in lung microvascular permeability caused by histamine, E. coli endotoxin, serotonin, microemboli, and several other substances.

The sheep lymph model is unique because it allows the investigator to collect lung lymph from unanesthetized animals. There may however be serious problems with the preparation. Taylor, Granger, and Brace[13] used the solute flux equation to estimate σ and PS for the lymph data from several tissues. They were unable to obtain reasonable results from sheep lymph data and observed that the problem occurred because PS (estimated from the lymph data) appeared to decrease when left atrial pressure was increased. One of the most important assumptions by investigators who have used the sheep lymph preparation is that it allows for the collection for almost pure lung lymph (about 95 percent pure). The finding of Taylor's group that the sheep lymph data appeared to be inconsistent with the simple equations of protein transport led some investigators to believe that the lymph was not pure. Recently we found that sheep have lymph vessels which transport peritoneal fluid into the caudal mediastinal lymph node and thus contaminate the lung lymph.[18] The contamination lymph flow rate is a significant fraction of the caudal mediastinal efferent flow (25 to 60 percent). The contaminating lymph protein concentration is approximately 60 to 70 percent of the plasma concentration and could well lead investigators to make incorrect conclusions based upon sheep lymph data.

Whether or not permeability is increased by pseudomonas, data from the study of Brigham and associates[17] shows that the pseudomonas-induced edema could well have been caused by elevated capillary hydrostatic pressure and lowered plasma oncotic pressure. When these investigators gave pseudomonas, Pc increased from 14.1 to 17.6 mmHg and the plasma protein concentration decreased from 6.7 to 5.75 g per dl. The decrease in plasma protein concentration would result in a decrease in πc of approximately 5 mmHg and a decrease in total safety factor against edema of about 7 to 8 mmHg.[6] The increase in Pc would also tend to produce edema. Additional data reported in Brigham's study demonstrated that edema developed only when Pc exceeded πc. This is completely consistent with the findings in several studies in which animals were not given any toxic agent. If the pseudomonas had significantly increased pulmonary vascular permeability, edema should have resulted at Pcs less than πc.

Changes in filtration Kf have also been used to detect a change in permeability. We have demonstrated in dog lungs that the filtration coefficient is increased by alloxan but not by histamine or E. coli endotoxin.[7]

Some investigators have used a multiple indicator dilution technique to detect permeability change in the lung. Basically two substances are injected into the right atrium: (1) an intravascular tracer and (2) a tracer which is permeable in the capillary membrane. As the tracers pass through the lung, some of the permeable tracer will diffuse into the tissue spaces so that it will appear in the systemic arterial blood in lower concentrations than a nonpermeable tracer. If the tracer molecules are properly chosen, it may be possible to estimate the permeability of the capillary membrane to the diffusible tracer. Unfortunately, it is necessary to develop a mathematical model to describe the tracer diffusion. Harris, Brigham, and Rowlett[19] used four different models to analyze the tracer curves of sheep given histamine. They found that three models indicated that permeability was increased with the histamine, but one showed no change. Another problem with the technique is that it has been used to estimate the permeability of very small molecules only (urea). It could be that some substances could change membrane permeability to small molecules without affecting the permeability to protein. Thus, even though small molecule permeability could be increased, it might have little or no affect upon lung fluid balance or the ability of the lung to withstand edema.

Changes in lung vascular permeability are difficult to detect even in laboratory animals. Investigators must choose between working with anesthetized animals which may have abnormal pulmonary permeability, or working with unanesthetized animals in which results of permeability tests are difficult to interpret. To date, studies which have indicated that increased permeability does occur with such agents as E. coli endotoxin, pseudomonas, and histamine have been done primarily on unanesthetized sheep. There is substantial evidence that these studies may have been misleading. Both the studies from anesthetized animals, as well as studies from unanesthetized animals, have demonstrated the role of increased capillary hydrostatic pressure and reduced plasma oncotic pressure in the development of pulmonary edema after the administration of toxic agents.

CONCLUSION

The Starling equation indicates that the plasma oncotic pressure should resist the formation of pulmonary edema. This fact has also been shown experimentally. The effectiveness of plasma oncotic pressure in resisting edema formation depends upon the permeability of the capillary membrane to protein. If permeability is significantly increased, as with alloxan, the plasma oncotic pressure becomes almost completely ineffective in resisting edema formation. However, there is little experimental evidence that the capillary membrane permeability is significantly increased in sepsis.

Once clinical pulmonary edema has developed, the process reverses slowly and unpredictably. The message for therapy is clear: *stay out of pulmonary edema.* Therapy can be most effective when the lung is not edematous if directed toward lowering capillary perfusion pressure and maintaining oncotic pressure.

REFERENCES

1. STARLING, EH: *On the absorption of fluids from the connective tissue spaces.* J Physiol 19:312, 1895.
2. GUYTON, AC, AND LINDSEY, AW: *Effect of elevated left atrial pressure and decreased plasma protein concentration on the development of pulmonary edema.* Circ Res 7:649, 1959.
3. MORRIS, AW, DRAKE RE, AND GABEL JC: *Comparison of microvascular filtration characteristics in isolated and intact lungs.* J Appl Physiol 48(3):438, 1980.
4. STAUB, NC: *The pathophysiology of pulmonary edema.* Human Path 1:419, 1970.
5. ERDMANN, AJ, ET AL: *Effect of increased vascular pressure on lung fluid balance in unanesthetized sheep.* Circ Res 37:271, 1975.
6. DRAKE, RE, SMITH, JH, AND GABEL, JC: *Estimation of the filtration coefficient in intact dog lungs.* Am J Physiol 238:H430, 1980.
7. DRAKE, RE, AND GABEL, JC: *Effect of histamine and alloxan on canine pulmonary vascular permeability.* Am J Physiol 239:196, 1980.
8. DRINKER, CK, AND FIELD, ME: *The protein content of mammalian lymph and the relation of lymph to tissue fluid.* Am J Physiol 97:32, 1931.
9. MEYER, BJ, MEYER, A, AND GUYTON, AC: *Interstitial fluid pressure vs. negative pressure in the lungs.* Circ Res 22:263, 1968.
10. GAAR, KA JR., ET AL: *Pulmonary capillary pressure and filtration coefficient in the isolated perfused lung.* Am J Physiol 213:910, 1967.
11. GABEL, JC, AND DRAKE, RD: *Pulmonary capillary pressure and permeability.* J Crit Care Med 7(3):92, 1979.
12. BRODY, JS, AND STEMMLER, EJ: *Differential reactivity in the pulmonary circulation.* J Clin Investigation 47:800, 1968.
13. TAYLOR, AE, GRANGER, DN, AND BRACE, RA: *Analysis of lymphatic protein flux data I: Estimation of the reflection coefficient and permeability surface area product for total protein.* Microvascular Res 13:297, 1977.

14. NORMAND, ICS, ET AL: *Permeability of lung capillaries and alveoli to non-electrolytes in the foetal lamb.* J Physiol 219:303, 1971.
15. PARKER, JC, ET AL: *The effect of fluid volume loading on exclusion of interstitial albumin of interstitial albumin and lymph flow in the dog lung.* Circ Res 45:440, 1979.
16. PARKER, JC, ET AL: *Vascular permeability and transvascular fluid and protein transport in the dog lung.* Circ Res 48:549, 1981.
17. BRIGHAM, KL, ET AL: *Increased sheep lung vascular permeability caused by pseudomonas bacteremia.* J Clin Invest 54:792, 1974.
18. DRAKE, R, ET AL: *Contamination of caudal mediastinal node efferent lymph in the sheep.* Accepted for publication by Am J Physiol.
19. HARRIS, TR, BRIGHAM, KL, AND ROWLETT, RD: *Pressure, serotonin, and histamine effects on lung multiple-indicator curves in sheep.* J Appl Physiol 44(2):245, 1978.

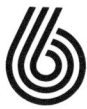

POST-TRAUMATIC RESPIRATORY FAILURE: ROLE OF FLUID THERAPY

George H. Rodman, Jr., M.D., and
Robert R. Kirby, M.D.

The fires of the raging controversy, "colloid versus crystalloid" have abated recently, but misinformation persists. Historically, there have been many swings of the pendulum. Shires' advocacy of balanced salts solutions during therapy of hemorrhagic shock was predicated on the loss of interstitial extracellular fluid volume which occurs simultaneously with blood loss. He never espoused the concept that Ringer's lactate solution was to be used as an alternate for blood. The original intent was that the crystalloid solution would leave—indeed was supposed to leave—the vascular space to replenish extracellular loss. However, Shires was misinterpreted, or perhaps overinterpreted, so that the misconceived sobriquet of "white blood" arose. Ringer's lactate certainly does not fulfill the requirements of oxygen carrying capacity and other functions as does blood. Over-enthusiastic use of balanced salt solutions caused widespread tissue edema. The lung obviously was a functional target and depository for such iatrogenic inundation. To make a difficult phenomenon impossible, detractors of balanced salt solution advocated that such pulmonary problems could be a routine consequence of resuscitation with crystalloid fluids. These individuals recommended plasma or albumin for their oncotic pressure sparing attributes. Later studies demonstrated this concept to be peculiarly unrewarding because of passage of albumin molecules into lung interstitial areas, and the grave economic consequences of such therapy. It is hoped that the pendulum is near mid-position now. Blood for blood loss, Ringer's lactate for extracellular deficits, in both proportional and not overly excessive degrees, should be the watchword of therapy. Drs. Rodman and Kirby explore these concepts with insight into their practical and esoteric scientific aspects in the following chapter.

Burnell R. Brown, Jr.

Modern therapy derived from study of pathophysiologic events associated with trauma and hemorrhagic shock emphasizes the simultaneous treatment priorities of controlling hemorrhage while replacing extracellular fluid (ECF) volume deficiencies. Preservation of organ system function is a direct benefit of adequate resuscitation. Recognition of respiratory insufficiency as a complication of major injury and its characterization as a form of pulmonary edema led to the belief that the margin of safety for fluid resuscitation was very narrow. Early understanding of the cause of post-traumatic pulmonary insufficiency linked this disease to the aggressive practice of vigorous fluid resuscitation of trauma patients. Published mortality rates exceeded 50 percent when respiratory failure occurred in victims of trauma.[1] Therapy of this disorder was initially based on time-honored principles which achieve reversal of *cardiogenic* pulmonary edema, that is, fluid restriction, osmotic, and diuretic agents. Most patients treated this way did not improve and mortality remained excessive.

Coupled with this therapeutic frustration was the apparent ambiguity of the term "fluid overload." Following complete resuscitation, some trauma patients showed signs of fluid excesses (peripheral edema, weight gain), but exhibited no signs of circulatory overload or pulmonary edema. Investigations aimed at unraveling the mysteries of tissue-vascular fluid exchange are still ongoing. But even without our understanding of principles governing tissue fluid exchange, mortality rates for post-traumatic pulmonary insufficiency are now substantially reduced.[2] Aggressive pulmonary therapy is ordinary physiotherapy, prolonged assisted ventilation, and airway pressure therapy in the form of continuous positive airway pressure (CPAP) and positive end expiratory pressure (PEEP). The key to success in treating this disorder seems to be the early institution of these modalities prior to severe deterioration of lung function.

As the disease has become more manageable, the controversy has intensified as to the ideal fluid regimen for prevention and treatment of post-traumatic pulmonary insufficiency. Most of the controversy centers around selection of a fluid regimen most likely to prevent accumulation of extravascular lung water, that is, crystalloid solution or colloid solutions. The following discussion reviews current data that supports selection of either regimen in the prevention and therapy of post-traumatic pulmonary insufficiency.

PATHOGENESIS

The adult respiratory distress syndrome (ARDS) which occurs in man after significant trauma is a nonspecific reaction of the lung. This syndrome is characterized by progressive hypoxemia in spite of inhalation of high concentrations of oxygen, but occurs without implicating a single cause. A number of eponyms have been applied to this syndrome in an attempt to allude to the apparent precipitating cause: shock lung, wet lung, post-traumatic lung, oxygen toxicity lung, respiratorory lung, congestive atelectasis, pump lung, DaNang lung, bronchopneumonia, pulmonary fat embolism syndrome, and finally, ARDS. But despite the presence or absence of specific etiologic factors, the same pathologic states occur in the pulmonary parenchyma. Clear separation of potential etiologic factors in the clinical situation is rarely possible. It is unlikely that there is any dominant single etiology, but rather combinations of factors, including shock, sepsis, overhydration, disseminated intravascular coagulation, oxygen toxicity, debris from massive transfusion, fat emboli, immunologic factors, aspiration, and central nervous system hypoxia. All are seemingly interrelated, though not always present in each case. Gross examination of these lungs at autopsy reveals hyperinflation saturation with fluid that oozes from cut surfaces of the lung. The primary increase in lung weight is due to interstitial edema.

Based on experimental studies of Moyer and coworkers[3] and Shires and associates[4], balanced electrolyte solutions, occasionally in large quantities, have become the mainstay of therapy for initial resuscitation of injured man. Depending on the depth and duration of the shock state, weight gain (10 to 15 percent above baseline) is obligatory and reflects the volume of fluid required to effect complete resuscitation. While such a practice may restore circulatory balance and improve immediate survival, many investigators blame "fluid overload" for the development of subsequent respiratory failure or shock lung. They reason that the initial shock state injures the lung and subsequent large quantities of fluid infusion enhance the formation of pulmonary edema. Such was the conclusion emerging from a conference on the pulmonary effects of nonthoracic trauma sponsored by the National Academy of Sciences.[5] Since many Vietnam combat casualties received large quantities of fluid, the apparently logical explanation was that fluid overload was the factor responsible for the pulmonary problems.

Subsequent investigators have demonstrated that shock per se probably does not cause shock lung. There is ample evidence that lung ischemia, unlike that which occurs in kidney, is well tolerated.[6] Additional conflicts in experimental results obtained from animal shock studies have subsequently been resolved by knowledge that species differences exist between nonvertebrates (i.e., dogs) and primates. The canine response to hemorrhage includes splanchnic (intestinal) and pulmonary congestion which is not seen in the primate. Although gross pulmonary changes do not seem to be a consequence of hemorrhagic shock in primates, electron microscopic studies have revealed ultrastructural pulmonary changes.[7] Moss and associates,[7] working with a baboon hemorrhagic shock model, demonstrated accumulation of sodium and water in the interstitial spaces of the lung. Further studies from these investigators demonstrated that saline infusions reverse these changes[8] in what at first glance seems to be paradoxical. The changes that were noted were not associated with any functional derangement.

One of the major mechanisms whereby fluid overload is thought to produce post-traumatic pulmonary insufficiency is related to the decrease in plasma oncotic pressure as a result of hemodilution following crystalloid resuscitation. Findings at the Vietnam Shock Unit confirmed a fall in plasma protein concentrations, but the most significant decrease occurred prior to resuscitation in the shock victims, with only a relatively slight additional drop following fluid infusion.[9] Furthermore, in trauma patients who develop respiratory distress syndrome, there is no apparent correlation between the amount of fluid given and the subsequent development of lung failure.[10] When massive inadvertent fluid overload occurs in trauma victims, the resultant pulmonary edema usually is readily reversible.

With the improved immediate management of trauma patients and specific attention directed toward respiratory care, severe manifestations of ARDS have developed less frequently in the immediate post-injury period. But the occurrence of ARDS many days or weeks following injury still is associated with a high mortality rate. Respiratory distress which develops during this late period inevitably follows secondary complications in the trauma patient, and is usually related to sepsis. The focus of sepsis is frequently intraperitoneal, although intrathoracic, major soft tissue, urinary tract, and venous sites are also possible sources. Many investigators have concluded that the unexpected appearance of pulmonary insufficiency after resuscitation from hemorrhagic shock following trauma is often the initial sign of severe infection.[6,11,12] Mortality rates in such patients with sepsis approach 70 percent.

Gump and associates[13] noted that in postoperative surgical patients, the degree of excess systemic fluid administration did not correlate with changes in lung water, but the presence of sepsis did. They concluded, therefore, that a change in vascular permeability was the primary factor that resulted in pulmonary edema. In those cases where sepsis has developed from wounds or peritonitis which precipitates respiratory distress, success in treating the respiratory distress is dependent upon effective control of the systemic infection. Currently, a number of investigators feel that the factors which predispose the injured patient to pulmonary failure are direct thoracic or pulmonary injury, sepsis, aspiration of gastric contents, head injury, and fat embolism. Of these factors, sepsis appears to jeopardize the patient's normal lung function most.[11]

There is no question that overenthusiastic administration of fluids will aggravate the underlying problem. If patients are given more fluid than they need, complications may develop which threaten survival. The primary question, however, is whether any protection of pulmonary function results from selection of the "ideal" fluid regimen for resuscitation of trauma victims.

THE "IDEAL" FLUID REGIMEN

There is little argument about the need to replace red blood cell loss with red blood cells. The ideal asanguinous fluid for extracellular fluid replacement, however, is controversial. Some investigators believe that one need only use a balanced salt solution to restore and maintain effective extracellular fluid volume.[14,15,16] Others feel strongly that the addition of colloid in the form of albumin is necessary in order to replenish and maintain plasma volume.[17,18] The latter groups cite the importance of maintaining plasma colloid oncotic pressure (COP) in order to minimize interstitial edema formation, expecially in the lung. Definite clinical evidence of the benefit of such therapy is lacking. In fact, recent clinical and experimental studies demonstrate that a balanced electrolyte solution, in addition to red blood cells, can be used safely regardless of the degree of volume deficit.[14,15,16] These studies have failed to show any detrimental pulmonary effects from such resuscitation. Proponents of crystalloid and colloid resuscitation regimens have found evidence supporting their position in reports of different animal experiments. Differing shock models, varied animal species, heterogenous protocols for fluid resuscitation, and the use of different endpoints to judge the effects of therapy have added to the confusion.

Moss and associates[8] demonstrated reversal of hemorrhagic shock-induced pulmonary ultrastructural changes when saline infusions were given. Gaisford, Pandey, and Jensen[19] demonstrated electron microscopic evidence of pronounced pulmonary interstitial edema in animals treated with Ringer's lactate, while animals treated with albumin infusions demonstrated almost no interstitial edema. A clue to the resolution of such conflicting data may be found in the different study designs related to resuscitation. Gaisford, Pandey, and Jensen[19] resuscitated animals according to the response of central venous pressure (CVP), not left ventricular filling pressure. The critical decision, therefore, may not lie in choosing the appropriate fluid, but rather in giving the appropriate amount of fluid to effect complete resuscitation.

The proponents of albumin solutions for resuscitation contend that these solutions provide comparable survival and improve cardiac and lung function while using lesser volumes. The suggested advantages of albumin are its tendency to increase the COP, remain in the vascular space, and minimize the amount of interstitial edema formation. These characteristics may be particularly important in the lung where increases in interstitial edema and extravascular lung water have been implicated as the etiology of respiratory distress syndrome following hemorrhagic shock and trauma.

In order to understand the dynamics of fluid exchange between pulmonary capillaries and the interstitium, concepts of pulmonary capillary pressure and capillary permeability require attention. Pulmonary fluid exchange is governed by the Starling equation:

$$Jv = Kf,c[Pc - Pt - \sigma(\pi c - \pi t)]$$

where Kf,c = capillary filtration coefficient, Pc = capillary hydrostatic pressure, Pt = tissue fluid hydrostatic pressure, σ = capillary membrane reflection coefficient to proteins, πc = oncotic pressure (COP), and πt = tissue fluid oncotic pressure.

Initially, clinicians were taught that capillaries were totally impermeable to plasma proteins. As such, forces tending to move fluid out of the capillary (hydrostatic) were exactly balanced by forces tending to keep fluid in the capillary (COP). Since the original assumption of protein impermeability now is known to be false,[20] the reflection coefficient has been added to account for the permeability of capillaries for plasma protein. If a membrane is impermeable to a solute, the reflection coefficient is 1; a freely difusable molecule such as water has a reflection coefficient of 0.

An increase in capillary hydrostatic pressure above its normal value alters other terms in the Starling equation. For example: (1) fluid movement across the membrane is increased; (2) as a result of this fluid egress, tissue fluid is diluted and tissue fluid oncotic pressure is decreased; (3) as fluid collects in the tissue, the tissue hydrostatic pressure increases; and (4) lymph flow increases.

Factors (2) and (3) above tend to offset the increased fluid movement across the capillary to the tissue. The ability of the lymphatic circulation to further compensate for the increased net fluid flux is called the *pulmonary safety factor*. Even though net fluid movement across the capillary occurs, opposing forces and the lymphatic safety factor may prevent the continuous accumulation of tissue fluid. The normal lymph flow (5 to 6 ml per 100 g lung tissue per hour) continuously decreases the tissue fluid oncotic pressure to a value approximately two-thirds of that of plasma.

Guyton and Lindsey[21] showed that the capillary hydrostatic pressure at which pulmonary edema develops is directly related to plasma COP. Although plasma COP can be decreased without producing pulmonary edema, subsequent increase in capillary hydrostatic pressure may predispose to pulmonary edema. Clinical estimates of pulmonary capillary hydrostatic pressure are derived from use of the Swan-Ganz catheter, that is, pulmonary artery occlusion pressure (PAOP). Guyton observed the appearance of pulmonary edema in dogs at a threshold left atrial pressure of 25 torr. He also found that reduction of COP in plasma by 50 percent resulted in a lower pulmonary edema threshold hydrostatic pressure of 11 to 13 torr. This observation was applied to the therapy of patients by Skillman, Parikl, and Tannenbaum,[22] who advocated raising plasma colloid levels with the infusion of colloid. The feeling persists that hypoalbuminemia (COP) favors the accumulation of fluid in the lung interstitium. In order for this to be true, two conditions must be present:

1. Pulmonary capillary membrane must be relatively impermeable to albumin under normal conditions.
2. No mechanism exists for the rapid removal of any albumin or fluid that enters the lung interstitium.

In fact, there is convincing evidence that neither of these conditions exists in the lung. Studies by Brigham and coworkers[23] and Zarins and associates[24] indicate that the difference in albumin concentration between plasma and pulmonary interstitium is quite small. In addition, both groups of investigators found that the pulmonary lymphatic system is efficient in washing out interstitial albumin (Fig. 1).

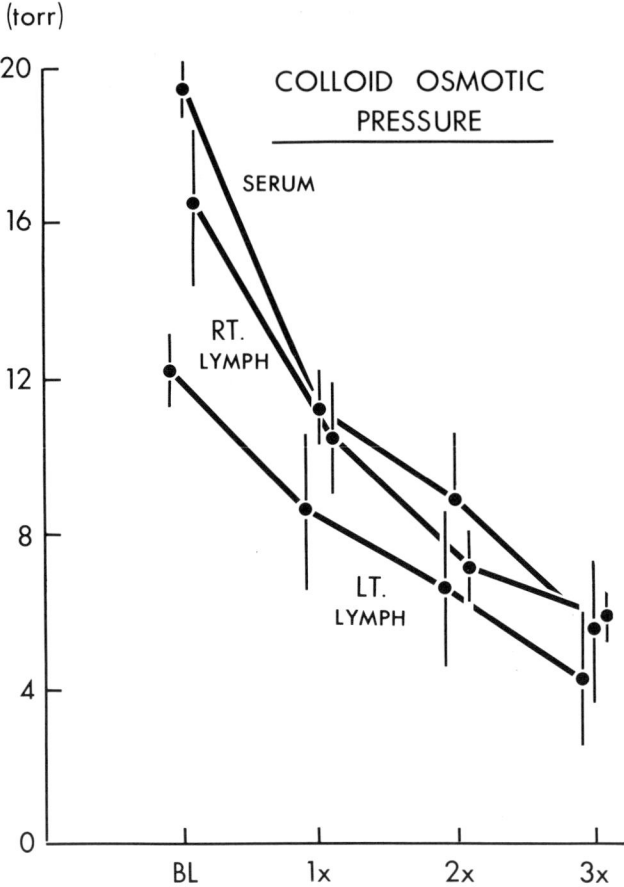

Figure 1. Effect of plasmapheresis on serum and right and left lymph oncotic pressures. Lung interstitial oncotic pressure is estimated in this model by collecting lymph in a subclavian vein pouch. As serum COP decreased, parallel decreases occur in both lung (right) and systemic (left) lymph oncotic pressures. (Adapted from Zarins et al.[24])

Furthermore, many investigators believe that pulmonary edema associated with injury and sepsis is caused by increased capillary permeability to protein.[20,23,25] Such a membrane change results in reduction of effective colloid oncotic pressure gradients across the membrane, and pulmonary edema develops if the safety factors (tissue hydrostatic pressure and lymph flow) cannot offset the increased net fluid flux to the interstitium. Such changes in permeability have been investigated by lymph protein flux analysis. Brigham, Woolverton, and Staub[26] produced an increased pulmonary vascular permeability by intravenous injection of pseudomonas bacteria in sheep. If left atrial pressure was elevated in any of these animals, massive fatal pulmonary edema ensued. They found that a similar infusion of pseudomonas bacteria into the right atrium of sheep caused a dramatic, prolonged, but reversible increase in pulmonary transvascular fluid and protein flow, independent of changes in vascular pressure. They concluded that since this increased flow amounted to a 10-fold increase in protein and fluid filtration, such changes would have occurred only if there was a change in the structure of the vascular wall, that is, an increase in permeability of the membrane. Moreover, in his review of pulmonary edema, Staub[20] pointed out that the lung is designed to compensate for fluid fluctuations in plasma proteins. As pulmonary capillary pressure increases, or plasma protein levels fall, more fluid moves through the capillary membrane into the interstitium. As long as fluid movement is moderate, it is readily mobilized by the lymphatics. The interstitial protein is washed out by the fluid movement, maintaining relatively normalized oncotic pressure gradients between vascular bed and interstitial space.

Zarins and associates[27] showed that the reduction of colloid oncotic pressure by plasmapheresis in baboons without increases in hydrostatic pressure (PAOP = <10 torr) did not lead to pulmonary edema. In a study by Rice and associates,[28] a 60 percent reduction in plasma COP (COP-PAOP gradient = 1 torr) following E. coli injection and plasmapheresis did not result in increased pulmonary edema measured by gravimetric techniques.

Confusion as to the effects of albumin on the injured lung is understandable when one considers there are minimal data available on the response of the normal pulmonary microcirculation to albumin infusions. Demling, Will, and Perea[29] used the chronic lung lymph fistula in sheep to describe the fate of albumin infusions. They concluded that in the normal lung, albumin infusion produces a significant increase in plasma COP, but also a transient rise in hydrostatic pressure, which appears to neutralize the increased plasma oncotic gradient. Interstitial COP increases following the increased plasma COP also tend to neutralize the effect of the latter. Because of these compensatory mechanisms of the pulmonary microcirculation, the absolute plasma COP after albumin infusion is an unreliable indicator of the state of extravascular (interstitial) lung water.

Holcroft and Trunkey[30] found no correlation between crystalloid or plasma resuscitation in the appearance of pulmonary edema during experimental shock in baboons. Both fluids were administered in amounts sufficient to restore pulmonary vascular pressures to normal. The lungs of animals resuscitated with blood and plasma were wetter than those animals resuscitated with Ringer's lactate. Although albumin extravasated into the interstitial tissues of the lung in both groups, this extravasation was greatest in animals resuscitated with plasma. A direct correlation between albumin extravasation and lung edema was noted. In a more recent study,[31] they demonstrated that in the early postresuscitation period extravasation of albumin into the pulmonary interstitium and increased extravascular lung water occurred transiently in crystalloid resuscitated animals. However, this excess lung water was mobilized and excreted by the first day after shock, emphasizing again the importance of lymph and albumin clearance (the pulmonary safety factor).

Further studies by Holcroft, Trunkey, and Carpenter[32] using both sheep and baboons showed that albumin extravasation occurs at different rates in various tissues. If their data can be extrapolated to man, albumin infusions administered to septic patients can be expected to prevent the formation of peripheral edema in skeletal muscle and possibly soft tissues such as skin and fat. Albumin infusions would not be expected to prevent edema in the lungs, heart, brain, or liver.

CLINICAL STUDIES

Luz and associates[18] concluded that decreasing COP associated with the use of albumin-free fluids during resuscitation substantially increases the risk of pulmonary edema. They reported that when the gradient between COP and PAOP fell below 9 torr, the risk of pulmonary edema was great. Unfortunately, in their studies pulmonary edema was defined by radiographic appearance and did not correlate well with alterations in arterial oxygen tension. Furthermore, their data suggests that decreasing COP-PAOP gradients are important in the development of pulmonary edema only when that decrease is caused by an increase in hydrostatic pressure, with or without concommitant changes in colloid oncotic pressure.

Lowe and associates[15] attempted to determine the relationship between resuscitation with either crystalloid or colloid solution and pulmonary function after trauma in man. The authors concluded that resuscitation with either crystalloid or colloid solution for acute trauma which required laparotomy did not produce significant differences between the two groups in terms of survival, incidence of pulmonary failure or postoperative pulmonary function. Although the majority of these patients were not massively injured (two-unit whole blood infusion requirement), the study showed that routine addition of albumin to the resuscitative regimen is unnecessary in such individuals undergoing emergency surgery for moderate trauma and hemorrhage.

Virgilio and associates[33] studied patients undergoing abdominal aortic reconstructive surgery who received either colloid or crystalloid fluid replacement in addition to washed packed red cells. Complete hemodynamic profiles were generated preoperatively, intraoperatively, and postoperatively. In addition, plasma COP was measured. The fluid administration rate during and after surgery was regulated to maintain pulmonary artery occlusion pressure ≤5 torr above baseline values. Intrapulmonary shunt and COP-PAOP gradients were calculated each time hemodynamic assessments were made. Both groups incurred positive fluid balance in the first 24 hours of therapy (day of surgery), but the crystalloid group gained twice as much weight over baseline (12 percent) as did the colloid group (6 percent). Despite this weight gain, there was no physiologic, radiographic, or clinical evidence of pulmonary edema. All patients were back to preoperative weight by the seventh day. Avoidance of any albumin in the crystalloid group resulted in a 40 percent decrease in COP and an 80 percent decrease in COP-PAOP from preoperative levels. Several patients in the crystalloid group had *negative* gradients, that is, PAOP > COP. (Fig. 2). Despite these changes in gradient, postoperative intrapulmonary shunts were identical in both groups and did not appear to be influenced by the type of fluid administered.

Perhaps the single most important factor responsible for the present controversy concerning the proper choice of fluid therapy is that past indirect estimates of lung hydration are not valid in clinical use. Lowenstein and associates[34] recently tested the reliability of arterial oxygen tension measurements in predicting changes in lung hydration. They showed that large changes in lung water are necessary for arterial oxygen tension to be affected. Total body weight is also inaccurate as a first approximation of lung hydration since the hydration state of muscle and subcutaneous tissue, which comprise 50 percent of body weight, may vary markedly for the same perturbation responsible for overhydration of the lung.

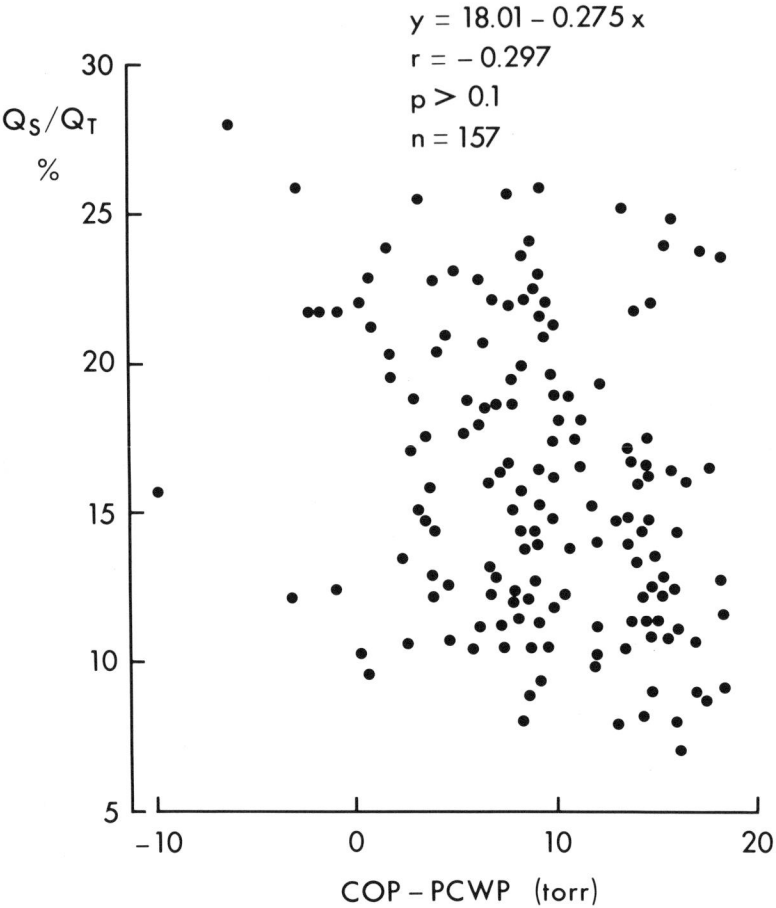

Figure 2. Relationship between fluid balance and shunt (Qs/Qt). During time when respiratory failure was being treated with PEEP, magnitude of positive fluid balance was not related to magnitude of intrapulmonary shunt. (From Gallagher, TJ and Civetta, JM American Society of Anesthesiology, Abstracts of Scientific Papers, 1976, with permission.)

Thermal-dye double indicator dilution techniques, aided by a microprocessor unit, give immediate bedside readout of extravascular lung water (EVLW) following injection of the indicators. Tranbaugh and associates[35] used the thermal-green dye double indicator dilution measurement of EVLW to follow daily lung water changes in seven severely burned adult patients resuscitated with crystalloid solutions alone. They concluded that massive crystalloid resuscitation while maintaining PAOP ≤15 torr does not cause an increase in EVLW during the first four days after thermal injury. EVLW actually decreased slightly in all patients despite marked weight gain, hypoproteinemia, and a negative plasma COP-PAOP gradient. EVLW did not correlate with plasma COP-PAOP gradient in either septic or nonseptic periods, even though in septic patients there was accumulation of lung water without any change in hydrostatic or oncotic pressures.

GUIDELINES FOR THERAPY

Improved survival from ARDS can be attributed partially to newer concepts of ventilator therapy and invasive cardiovascular monitoring.[2] Titration of fluid administration rates to assure optimal oxygen delivery requires reliance on pulmonary artery catheter generated data such as PAOP, stroke volume, (SV) and cardiac output (CO). Simultaneous increased "titration" of PEEP to yield a reduced intrapulmonary shunt has led to reduced mortality due to ARDS.[36] No matter what fluid regimen is chosen, careful attention to optimization of preload factors (PAOP) is the first step toward establishing optimal hemodynamic function during therapy for ARDS. A restrictive fluid regimen aimed at "drying the lungs" may result in a suboptimal hemodynamic profile that "drys" the organism with sacrifice of other organ function (renal and hepatic). Conversely, a fluid regimen aimed at achieving optimal cardiac function without incurring excess pulmonary vascular hydrostatic pressure (PAOP 14 to 17 torr) is both rational and safe. However, pressures in the pulmonary vascular bed are subject to occasional errors in measurement or interpretation.

Normally, PAOP measurements are made at end-expiration when intrathoracic and pleural pressure are at their baseline values. At this point, PAOP approximates left atrial pressure. But if at end-expiration, PEEP prevents the return of alveolar pressure and pleural pressure to baseline, then the *true* (transmural) atrial filling pressure is the difference between measured intravascular pressure (PAOP) and extravascular pressure (pleural pressure). Although relatively safe and reliable methods for measuring pleural pressure are available, appropriate interpretation must await a clearer understanding of regional variations.

PEEP can also influence the accuracy of interpretation of PAOP by its effect on the pulmonary circulation. Alveolar pressure can be transmitted to the pulmonary capillaries and cause them to collapse. The pressure measurement on the arterial end of the collapsed vessel clearly is not equal to the pressure at the distal end, but instead reflects the collapsing pressure, in this case alveolar pressure, or PEEP. Such aberrations occur consistently above 25 cm water pressure PEEP. A 5 cm water increase in PEEP which produces a similar elevation in PAOP probably means PAOP measurements are tracking alveolar, not atrial pressure. Kirby and associates have shown that for PEEP up to 25 cm water pressure, the change in PAOP "on" and "off" PEEP can be predicted from the following formula:

$$PAOP(torr) = 0.14(PEEP\ cm\ H_2O) + 1.5$$

Another method proposed to detect the alveolar pressure artifact in PAOP measurement at high levels of PEEP requires repeating PAOP measurements off PEEP. Some reservations must exist in interpreting PAOP on and off PEEP since the two measurements probably reflect separate and unrelated hemodynamic relationships. Sudden cessation of PEEP may result in acute increases in preload volume and filling pressure (off PEEP) leaving little, if any, resemblance to preload factors while on PEEP. After intravascular volume expansion, one frequently observes minimal changes in PAOP, even though PAOP readings on PEEP may be high (15 to 20 torr) prior to infusion. Simultaneously, however, CO may increase significantly. This effect seems to be typical of patients treated with high levels of PEEP, and who have large measured differences (≥ 5 torr) in PAOP on and off PEEP. The consistency of this response is strong presumptive evidence for hypovolemia.

CONCLUSION

Fluid administration to the trauma patient must be in accordance with previously stated goals which include: (1) maintenance and replacement of blood volume and interstitial fluid, (2) correction of existing deficits, and (3) anticipation of additional third space losses. Patients often require larger than expected quantities of fluid in addition to blood replacement if the shock state has been prolonged. Rarely do our estimates of fluid deficit correlate with the actual amounts ultimately required. Anatomic expansion of the ECF (weight gain) is a physiologic necessity if the *functional* ECF deficit is to be completely restored. Controversy arises when discussion turns to the necessity for protein (albumin) replacement. Volume for volume, protein-containing solutions will restore intravascular volume to a greater extent than will balanced electrolyte solutions. Resuscitation to precise physiologic endpoints with either solution requires a volume of balanced salt solution 2 to 4 times that of protein-containing solutions. Resuscitation with protein-containing solutions has been suggested to minimize the accumulation of intestinal pulmonary edema and the occurrence of ARDS associated with resuscitation following traumatic shock. Neither experimental nor clinical studies demonstrate the protective pulmonary effect of albumin compared with balanced electrolyte solution. Since no clear physiologic advantage of albumin solution can be shown, a rational choice of resuscitative fluids should consider economic factors; albumin-containing solutions cost about 30 times as much per liter as balanced-salt solutions.

Overall diagnostic and therapeutic measurements, including adequate cardiorespiratory monitoring and specific treatment such as PEEP for respiratory failure have become widespread. As a result, neither the incidence nor the severity of respiratory failure carries the morbid significance that it did a few short years ago. Since the manipulation of oncotic pressure is an ancillary supportive maneuver at best, it is probable that the availability of proven effective diagnostic and therapeutic measures has eliminated the necessity for the as yet unproven efficacy of colloids. The so-called colloid-crystalloid controversy is simply no longer relevant. Comprehensive care, including total ventilatory support, nutrition, and attention to all major organ systems, is the most significant factor in improving survival.

REFERENCES

1. MOORE, FD, ET AL: *Post-traumatic Pulmonary Insufficiency.* WB Saunders, Philadelphia, 1969.
2. CIVETTA, JM, ET AL: *Aggressive treatment of acute respiratory insufficiency.* South Med J 69:749, 1976.
3. MOYER, CA, ET AL: *Burn shock and extravascular sodium deficiency—Treatment with Ringer's solution with lactate.* Arch Surg 90:799, 1965.
4. SHIRES, GT, ET AL: *Fluid therapy in hemorrhagic shock.* Arch Surg 88:688, 1964.
5. EISEMAN, B AND ASHBAUGH, D (EDS): *Pulmonary effects of non-thoracic trauma.* J Trauma 8:625, 1968.
6. COLLINS, JA: *The causes of progressive pulmonary insufficiency in surgical patients.* J Surg Res 9:685, 1969.
7. MOSS, GS, ET AL: *Effect of hemorrhagic shock on pulmonary interstitial sodium distribution in the primate lung.* Ann Surg 177:211, 1973.

8. Moss, GS, ET AL: *The effect of saline resuscitation on pulmonary sodium and water distribution.* Surg Gynecol Obstet 136:934, 1973.
9. Bredenberg, CE: *Acute respiratory distress syndrome.* Surg Clin North Am 54:1043, 1974.
10. Shires, GT, ET AL: *Shock.* WB Saunders, Philadelphia, 1973.
11. Horovitz, JH, ET AL: *Pulmonary response to major injury.* Arch Surg 108:349, 1974.
12. Vito L, ET AL: *Sepsis presenting as acute respiratory insufficiency.* Surg Gynecol Obstet 138:896, 1974.
13. Gump, FE, ET AL: *Water balance and extravascular lung water: Measurements in surgical patients.* Am J Surg 119:515, 1970.
14. Moss, GS, ET AL: *A comparison of asanguinous fluid and whole blood in the treatment of hemorrhagic shock.* Surg Gynecol Obstet 129:1247, 1969.
15. Lowe, RJ, ET AL: *Crystalloid vs. colloid in the etiology of pulmonary failure after trauma: A randomized trial in man.* Surgery 81:676, 1977.
16. Moss, GS: *An argument in favor of electrolyte solution for early resuscitation.* Surg Clin North Am 52:3, 1972.
17. Skillman, JJ: *The role of albumin and oncotically active fluids in shock.* Crit Care Med 4:55, 1976.
18. Luz, PL, ET AL: *Pulmonary edema related to changes in colloid osmotic and pulmonary artery wedge pressure in patients after acute myocardial infarction.* Circulation 51:350, 1975.
19. Gaisford, WD, Pandey, N, AND Jensen, CG: *Pulmonary changes in treated hemorrhagic shock: II. Ringer's lactate solution versus colloid infusion.* Am J Surg 124:738, 1972.
20. Staub, NE: *Pulmonary edema.* Physiol Rev 54:687, 1971.
21. Guyton, AC AND Lindsey, AW: *Effect of elevated left atrial pressure and decreased plasma protein concentration on the development of pulmonary edema.* Circ Res 7:649, 1959.
22. Skillman, JJ, Parikl, BM, AND Tanenbaum, BJ: *Pulmonary venous admixture: Improvement with albumin and diuretics.* Am J Surg 119:440, 1970.
23. Brigham, KL, ET AL: *Increased sheep lung vascular permeability caused by pseudomonas bacteremia.* J Clin Invest 54:792, 1974.
24. Zarins, CK, ET AL: *Role of lymphatics in preventing hypooncotic pulmonary edema.* Surg Forum 27:257, 1976.
25. Achanar, BM, ET AL: *Pulmonary complications of burns: The major threat to the burn patient.* Ann Surg 177:311, 1973.
26. Brigham, KL, Woolverton, WC, AND Staub, NC: *Reversible increase in pulmonary vascular permeability after pseudomonas aeruginosa bacteremia in unanesthetized sheep.* Chest 65 (Suppl 4): 51, 1974.

27. Zarins, CK, et al.,: *Lymph and pulmonary response isobaric reduction in plasma oncotic pressure.* Circ Res 43:925, 1979.
28. Rice, CL, et al: *The effect of sepsis and reduced colloid osmotic pressure on pulmonary edema.* J Surg Res 27:347, 1979.
29. Demling, RH, Will, JA, and Perea, A: *Effect of albumin infusion on pulmonary microvascular fluid and protein transport.* J Surg Res 27:321, 1979.
30. Holcroft, JW and Trunkey, DD: *Extravascular lung water following hemorrhagic shock in the baboon: Comparison between resuscitation with Ringer's lactate and plasmanate.* Ann Surg 180:408, 1974.
31. Holcroft, JW, and Trunkey, DD: *Pulmonary extravasation of albumin during and after hemorrhagic shock in baboons.* J Surg Res 18:91, 1975.
32. Holcroft, JW, Trunkey, DD, and Carpenter, MA: *Extravasation of albumin in tissues of normal and septic baboons and sheep.* J Surg Res 26:341, 1979.
33. Virgilio, RW, et al: *Crystalloid vs. colloid resuscitation: Is one better?* Surgery 85:129, 1979.
34. Lowenstein, E, et al: *Lung and heart water accumulation associated with hemodilution.* Bibl Haemotol 41:190, 1975.
35. Tranbaugh, RF, et al.,: *Lung water changes after thermal injury.* Ann Surg 192:479, 1980.
36. Kirby, RR, Civetta, JM, Gallagher, TJ, et al.: *The effect of PEEP on pulmonary capillary wedge pressure* (abstr). Scientific Papers 1976 ASA Annual Meeting, 229, 1976.

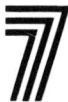

BALANCED SALT SOLUTIONS AS RENAL PROPHYLAXIS

Charles A. Baxter, M.D.

Dr. Baxter discusses the issue of renal function preservation during shock resuscitation. Concerning olguria, I recall the reality of the post-operative patient with renal shutdown. It is now well recognized that the cause of this condition was the lack of adequate replacement of extracellular fluid. When urinary volume decreased as a normal response to fluid depletion, fluids were restricted even more, giving a coup de gras to renal integrity. This is a problem rarely seen today, with liberalized use of saline or balanced salt solutions.

Polyuric renal failure, or high output failure, is more common in our era than is oliguric failure. It can be seen with shock, infection, and as a complication of certain drug administration. Dr. Baxter discusses this disease process and suggests means to prevent or lessen the likelihood of its occurrence.

Burnell R. Brown, Jr.

Acute, recoverable loss of renal function is a formidable complication in surgical patients. During the last 15 years, the incidence of classic oliguric acute renal failure resulting from severe shock and blood transfusion reactions has decreased dramatically as a result of rapid transportation and prompt care of the severely injured, the treatment of shock, and the intraoperative and postoperative management of fluid volume of both trauma patients and those undergoing elective surgery. The use of balanced salt solutions in all these areas of patient care delivery has been largely responsible for reducing renal complications.

The incidence has been reduced from approximately 1 in 200 patients to 1 in 600 patients treated surgically for severe injury. The overall incidence is less dramatically reduced, since over one third of the cases in the recovery period occur as a result of infection, antibiotic administration, or hematologic complications.

There is increasing recognition of less severe types of acute renal insufficiency that may complicate the clinical course of surgical illnesses. Nonoliguric acute renal failure has become the most common clinical form of renal damage diagnosed, and less severe clinical states that are important in the total management of surgical patients have recently been described.[1]

Although the pathophysiology of acute renal insufficiency is incompletely understood, the incidence and severity of damage can be decreased by constant awareness of the etiologic factors and effective use of preventive measures throughout the course of treatment of surgical patients.

PREVENTION OF ACUTE RENAL INSUFFICIENCY

The majority of cases of acute renal insufficiency occur in association with injuries or operations producing severe or protracted blood loss or shock. The highest incidence is observed in cases of extensive intra-abdominal or retroperitoneal injury, major blood vessel injury, and trauma affecting multiple systems. Less well recognized are cases of incipient blood loss or incomplete replacement of volume deficits in which compensatory mechanisms obscure the signs of hypovolemia and protracted renal ischemia. The use of vasopressors in the initial resuscitation of patients with shock due to blood loss results in a very high incidence of renal complications, so their use has been virtually eliminated in the management of hemorrhagic shock. Less frequently, renal insufficiency results from massive hemolysis of transfusion incompatibility, or myoglobinuria from extensive muscle damage.

Many cases of acute renal failure in these categories can be prevented by several methods now routinely employed in the management of shock, trauma, and transfusion reactions. These include the use of balanced salt solutions in addition to blood replacement in the initial resuscitation in hemorrhagic shock, the recognition and replacement of all fluid volume deficits resulting from injury to various organ systems, and an effective means of decreasing renal tubular metabolism with regional hypothermia when the rates of fluid loss exceed the capacity for immediate replacement.

Hemorrhagic shock has been shown to be associated with the functional loss of extracellular fluid.[2] The initial resuscitation of most shock patients is begun with the administration of approximately 2000 ml balanced salt solution, permitting time for the acquisition of type-specific blood in the majority of severe cases, and allowing accurate crossmatching in most cases.

The use of balanced salt solution initially in resuscitation in shock serves a dual function in correcting the isotonic sodium ion depletion resulting from movement of sodium into cells, and often alleviating the shock by temporary plasma volume expansion for a period sufficient to permit typing and crossmatching of blood, thereby reducing the incidence of transfusion incompatibility.

Rapid and complete blood replacement is imperative in the management of trauma and shock. Equally important, however, is the replacement of the isotonic fluid sequestrations that occur as a result of soft tissue injury. Sequestration of large quantities of extracellular fluid results from the contusion of large muscle masses, soft tissue damage occurring with long bone fractures, or prolonged interruption of vascular supply to the extremities. Both direct trauma and operative injury to visceral organs, particularly the small bowel, produce rather large intraluminal and intramural collections of extracellular fluid, in addition to the chemical peritonitis produced by the intra-abdominal spillage of digestive fluids. It is often difficult to estimate accurately the volume of fluid lost in these situations. The return of normal blood pressure and pulse rate in patients in the supine position may occur even though replacement is deficient by as much as a liter of blood or several liters of extracellular fluid. The hourly monitoring of urine volumes and central venous pressure after initial resuscitation following fluid replacement under anesthesia, and in the postoperative state, is necessary to evaluate the adequacy of fluid replacement.

The most important treatment measure in hemolytic transfusion is to establish the presence of adequate urinary volume at the time of the reaction. An established urine output at the time of transfusion reaction markedly reduces the incidence of heme pigment precipitation and the formation of protein casts in the renal tubules. Adequate urine output is enhanced by the administration of 1 liter of sixth-molar sodium lactate given rapidly, followed by a second liter at a slower rate to maintain a urine volume of over 100 ml per hour until hemoglobinuria lessens. Mannitol in doses of 12.5 g per hour is reserved for those cases in which such diuresis is not produced by the administration of additional alkalinizing volume. In 28 consecutive cases of reaction to mismatched transfusion in patients with adequate urinary output, no renal failure occurred.

Myoglobinuria occurring as the initial manifestation of severe muscle damage or, later, as a result of prolonged interruption of major arterial supply to large muscle masses, has been associated with a high incidence of renal failure. Employing sufficient isotonic fluid volume therapy to replace the losses of fluid occurring in the damaged area, alkalinizing the urine with molar sodium bicarbonate in sufficient quantities to produce an alkaline pH and prevent the precipitation of acid hematin, and the administration of mannitol at a rate of 12.5 g per hour, have virtually eliminated renal failure as a complication of this entity.

The highest incidence of renal insufficiency occurs when there is severe or continuing blood loss. Renal ischemia, and particularly cortical hypoxia, may be severe and prolonged. Evidence of the efficacy of protecting the kidney from ischemia damage by hypothermia is well documented.[3] Hypothermia is used during surgery when shock is severe or prolonged, or when it recurs during a surgical procedure, and in other special instances, such as temporary clamping of the aorta or renal arteries.

When laparotomy is required, sufficient protection can be afforded the kidney by regional hypothermia carried out by sluicing the peritoneal cavity with a cold isotonic solution (4°C) at 1 to 1½ hour intervals throughout the operative procedure. Approximately 2 liters is poured into the open abdominal cavity at logical intervals during the procedure; the solution is allowed to remain in contact with the upper retroperitoneal area for five minutes, and then withdrawn by suction.

With this method, a rapid decrease in the core temperature of the kidney occurs when renal blood flow is significantly decreased (Fig. 1). Patients with hypotension and some decrease in renal blood are

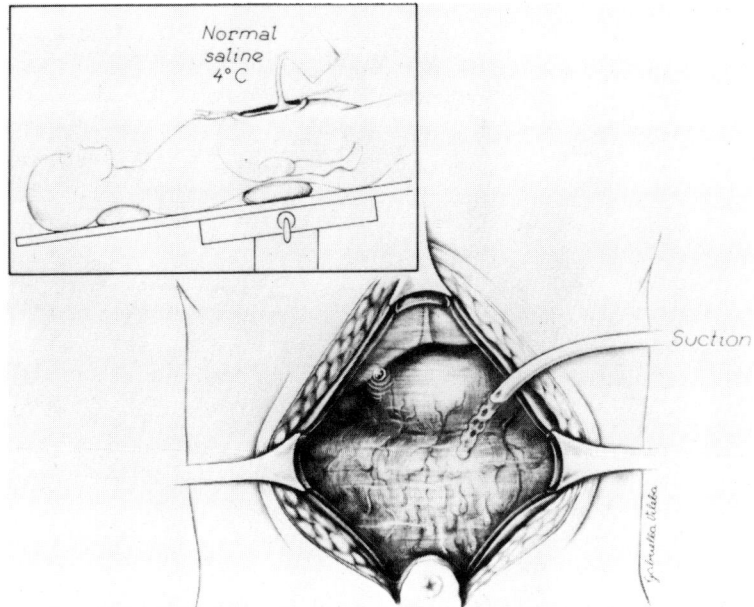

Figure 1. Technique of regional abdominal hypothermia. One or two liters of 4°C isotonic saline (refrigerator temperature) are slurred onto the upper retroperitoneal area. The operating table is lowered to keep the solution over the kidney fossa for 3 to 5 minutes.

cooled less rapidly; significant cooling does not occur when renal blood flow is normal. No detrimental effect on the kidney itself has been seen, nor have postoperative complications been observed with extensive use of this procedure.

Significant protection is afforded an ischemic kidney by reducing the intrarenal temperature by 8 to 10°C (Fig. 2). This effective, safe, and rapid method of cooling is readily available in all operating rooms.[1]

More recently, defective oxygen delivery at the tissue level in routine management of patients has been implicated in tissue damage. The quantity of oxygen delivered to the tissues is dependent upon the hemoglobin concentration, cardiac output, and the ability of the blood to release oxygen at the tissue level. Deficits of 2,3-diphosphoglycerate (2,3-DPG) in stored blood, hypothermia, and alkalosis result in the shift to the left of the oxygen dissociation curve, and hence decreased tissue oxygen delivery. In recent experiments by Canizaro and associates,[2] the progressive addition of anemia, 2,3-DPG defi-

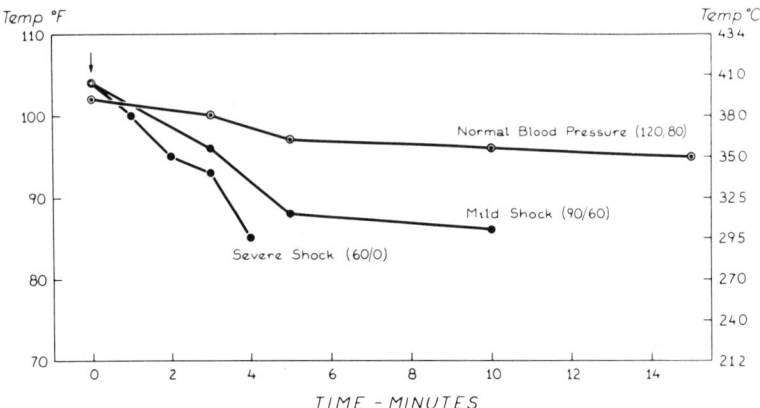

Figure 2. Regional hypothermia in patients. Renal core temperature measured in 10 patients with varying degrees of hypotension shock during laporatomy for trauma, compared with 10 elective surgical patients with normal blood pressure.

ciency, hypothermia, and respiratory alkalosis resulted in a progressive shift to the left of the oxygen dissociation curve. The P_{50} in these experimental animals was observed to be below the critical tissue oxygen tension of most of the vital organ systems, including the kidney.

Similar changes may be prevented clinically by the use of whole blood preserved by citrate-phosphorus-dextrose (CPD) anticoagulants, which maintain a satisfactory level of 2,3-DPG for seven days. Fresh blood should be given as often as possible, preferably every third unit. Maintaining a normal core temperature with external heating devices and warming of blood and the intravenous fluids decreases this component of the oxygen dissociation curve shift. Nonhyperventilation techniques are currently being more widely employed in patients, and intraoperative monitoring of pH and blood gases used as a guide to preventing significant pH changes.

Potent tubular blocking agents (furosemide, ethacrynic acid) have been recommended for routine use in traumatized and surgical patients.[4] Since the incidence of renal damage associated with emergency surgery is less than 1 percent, and is even lower in elective surgery, the use of such drugs seems unwise in some circumstances. For example, the assessment of circulatory stability under anesthesia is difficult when the rate of urine formation, a good index of organ perfusion, is no longer reliable. With the use of these diuretics, urine may be produced when cardiac output is diminished or one of the aforementioned tissue-oxygen delivery factors is deficient.[5]

Anesthetic agents such as methoxyflurane (Penthrane) are now known to be nephrotoxic when used in high concentrations, over long periods, or in patients with diminished renal reserve (over 50 years of age).[6]

RENAL RESPONSES FOLLOWING SURGERY AND TRAUMA

The spectrum of renal damage following surgery or trauma can be appreciated from studies that identify normal and abnormal responses to surgery. In a recent clinical study of 40 trauma patients selected for study from 1000 cases of trauma requiring operation, serial renal function studies were carried out under conditions that were as closely controlled as possible in such a study.[7] The study showed that graded renal damage occurs in association with systemic injury, and that identification of patients with subclinical, mild, and severe renal damage is important in their postsurgical care.

Subclinical Renal Damage Following Injury and Shock

Comparison of the renal function studies of the 40 patients in the study cited above identified a group (30 patients) who were considered to show the characteristic renal response to trauma, eight patients with subclinical renal function, and two patients with nonoliguric progressive azotemia. The patients were divided into two groups according to their blood urea nitrogen values (Fig. 3). As would be expected on the basis of the selection criteria from the group, the glomerular filtration rate differed between the groups (Fig. 4). Cardiac output between the two groups was not significantly different.

Urea clearance (C_{urea}), another clearance principally related to filtration, was depressed in both groups initially, with a rapid return to normal and above in the characteristic group, and slowly toward normal in the dysfunction group. Urine-plasma urea ratios and osmolar clearances (C_{osm}) differed between the two groups only after 12 hours following admission. The urine-plasma urea ratios for both groups are shown in Figure 5. Tubular reabsorption of water (TC_{H_2O}) was significantly different between the two groups only 18 and 24 hours after admission. The trend in group 1 was toward excretion of

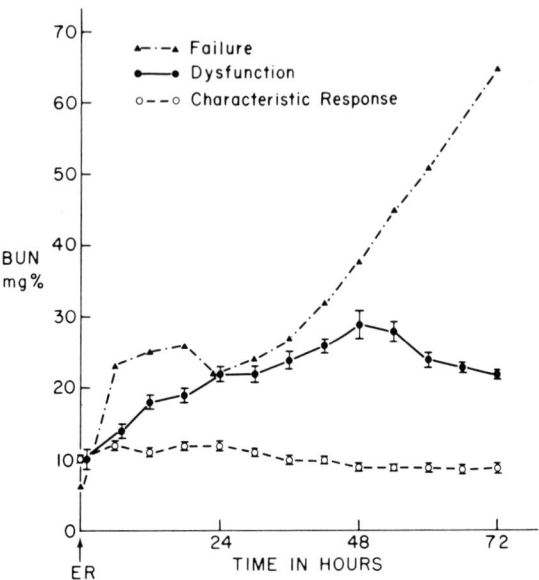

Figure 3. Renal function after trauma: blood urea nitrogen values.

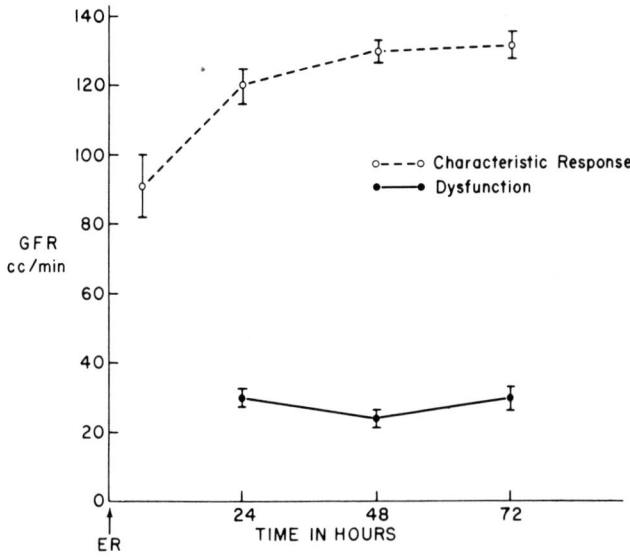

Figure 4. Renal function after trauma: glomerular filtration rate determined by iothalamate ^{125}I constant infusion method.

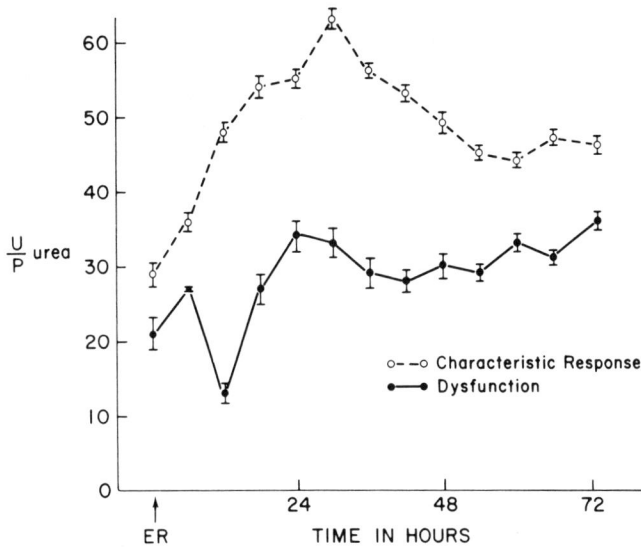

Figure 5. Renal function after trauma: urine to plasma-urea ratio.

free water, while the trend in the dysfunction group was toward continued retention of free water.

There were no discernible differences between the two groups in age, type of injury, length of hypotensive episodes, fluid and electrolyte requirements for resuscitation, postoperative intravenous fluid administration, positive-pressure ventilation, nephrotoxic antibiotics, blood volume, urine volume, or arterial oxygen concentration of pH.

Sodium clearances in the two groups were similar for 12 hours following admission. Then sodium clearance in the second group fell (Fig. 6). Postoperative sodium balance represented by the difference between daily sodium intake and urinary sodium excretion was different in the two groups. Group 1 showed positive sodium balance during the first day, positive balance during the second day, and negative balance during the third day. In group 2, the dysfunction group, increasing sodium retention occurred during each of the three days of study. The documentation of this renal abnormality, undetectable by usual clinical criteria for diagnosis, explains the tendency toward circulatory overloads encountered in patients who have had severe stress when large quantities of fluid become available for excretion.

These studies show that neither azotemia nor elevated creatinine is an inevitable consequence of severe tissue injury, and that other fac-

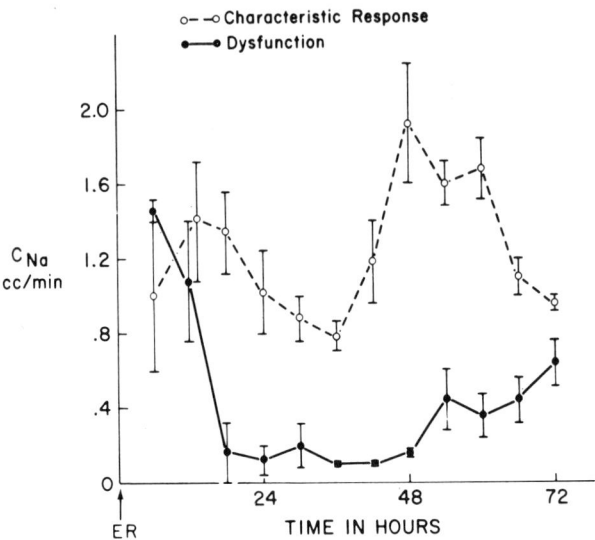

Figure 6. Renal function after trauma: sodium clearance.

tors are operative in the injured patient who exhibits such changes. Flear and Clarke[8] demonstrated that patients given transfusions lost less nitrogen in the period following injury than similarly injured patients who were not transfused. It is not surprising that metabolism and nitrogen excretion are inversely related to the adequacy of resuscitative therapy. The patient with the greatest catabolic response has sustained a more severe injury than one who does not demonstrate such changes. Flear and Clarke also demonstrated that transfused patients have negative sodium balance after the first day, as did group 1 patients in this study. The nature of the differences and the response of the two groups of patients may lie in individual patient differences and in currently unquantifiable differences in the degree of primary injury.

The earliest possible restoration of circulating volume with electrolyte solutions and blood, combined with the definitive treatment of injury, should decrease the degree of secondary systemic injury. Conversely, even minimal persistent elevations of blood urea nitrogen are uniformly associated with significant renal dysfunction and sodium and water retention. Identification of the more severely injured patient in the early postoperative phase can readily be accomplished by serial evaluation of renal metabolism of urea or sodium. Such identification should lead to meticulous supportive care of the general metabolic reserve of the more severely injured patient, in whom renal reserve is diminished and further insults are poorly tolerated.

High-Output (Nonoliguric) Renal Failure

Progressive uremia occurring without a period of oliguria and accompanied by a daily urine volume of greater than 1000 to 1500 ml per day is now recognized as the most frequently diagnosed clinical variant of renal failure occurring in association with surgery and trauma. Recognition of this entity has established the variable severity of renal damage and has indicated the frequency with which some renal damage occurs as a complication of trauma, shock, infection, and nephrotoxic drug administration.

High-output renal failure is from 5 to 10 times more frequent than oliguric renal failure. The special importance of high-output renal failure lies in the fact that it is generally a milder form of renal insufficiency, which if diagnosed early and managed correctly, is usually not fatal. Mean values for the typical clinical course of such patients are shown in Figure 7. There is mounting azotemia for a mean of 10 days, with progressive decrease toward normal for the next 10 to 12 days. The azotemia is accompanied by urine volumes which generally increase daily, reaching their height at the peak of azotemia, then gradually returning to normal range. In a series of 27 trauma patients, the spectrum varied from very mild elevations of blood urea nitrogen of 50 to 70 mg per 100 ml, to severe azotemia of 240 to 250 mg per 100 ml urea nitrogen. The wide spectrum of the severity of damage in this type of renal failure suggests that it is a less severe form of a similar process that produces oliguric renal failure.

Serial measurements of blood urea nitrogen, potassium, carbon dioxide combining power, and chlorides permit intelligent chemical and fluid management with a much greater latitude because of the large obligatory daily urine volume excretion.

The mortality rate for high output acute renal failure in this series was 18.5 percent, compared with the extremely high mortality for oliguric renal failure.[9] The deaths were thought to result from complications of the injury and are, in general, not related to the renal failure. However, infection is the most frequent cause of death in these patients, as well as in patients with oliguric renal insufficiency.

This type of renal failure is not specific for traumatic injury. It may occur in association with elective surgical procedures, in nonelective

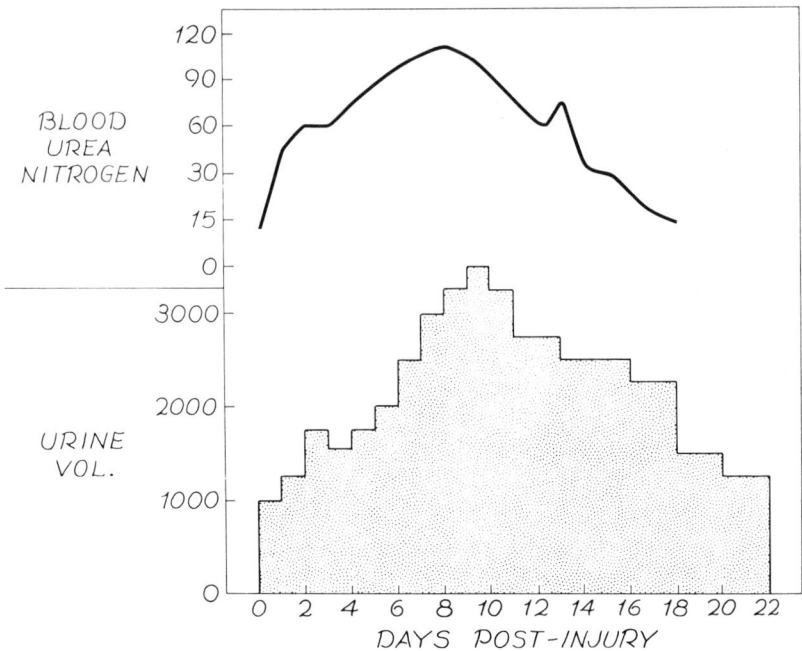

Figure 7. Mean values for daily urine volumes and blood urea nitrogen (BUN) concentrations for 27 patients with high output renal failure.

surgical illnesses, usually involving infection or shock, and with the administration of nephrotoxic agents such as methoxyflurane, outdated tetracycline, and aminoglycosides.[10,11]

Increased recognition of this entity has resulted in the implication of many nephrotoxic factors that produce some degree of renal damage. Fortunately, most of these agents are weak (mild) nephrotoxic agents, and careful use minimizes this danger. For example, lowering the daily dose of gentamicin from 4 g per kg body weight per day after 48 hours of use to one half of that dose virtually eliminates nephrotoxicity.

Oliguric Renal Failure

Oliguric renal failure is the most severe renal lesion in the spectrum of renal damage. Profound oliguria (urine volumes of 100 to 200 ml per day) does not usually occur abruptly, except in instances of transfusion reaction or myoglobinuric nephrosis.[12] Most often urine volumes are between 400 and 500 ml per 24 hours on the first day, then progressively decrease over the next 2 to 4 days, becoming fixed at 50 to 200 ml per day. Early diagnosis (using the blood-urine urea ratio) is important to prevent excessive fluid overloads, avoid potassium administration, and curtail protein intake to minimize the rise in potassium and urea which usually occurs very rapidly in the early oliguric period.

Prophylactic dialysis offers great advantage in salvage of patients compared with dialysis undertaken on the basis of clinical deterioration or chemical signs of severe uremia, acidosis, or hyperkalemia.

The choice of dialysis procedure should be individualized. Peritoneal dialysis is preferable when abdominal surgery has not been performed. It is also employed preferentially when the circulation is unstable, since demodialysis under these circumstances often produces uncorrectable shock. Hemodialysis is selected for all patients with previous abdominal surgery and for those in whom intra-abdominal complications are suspected. Arteriovenous shunts (Scribner) are placed 12 to 24 hours before the initial dialysis procedure, and regional heparinization is employed when bleeding may be produced by anticoagulation.

Prophylactic dialysis, using ultrafiltration, permits greater fluid intake, since the excess fluid may be removed by daily dialysis. Fluid volumes of 1000 to 1200 ml per day are utilized for the administration of essential amino acid solutions and large glucose and insulin intakes. Total intake of 2000 calories per day suppresses the rate of blood urea nitrogen rise in the plasma, presumably by decreasing gluconeogenesis from endogenous protein.

Awareness of the fact that acute renal failure patients seldom show the usual diagnostic signs of infection, inflammation, or pain will often permit early diagnosis of intervening complications. For example, perforated ulcers occur without pain, and peritonitis may manifest only by ileus.

Surgical procedures are hazardous in patients with acute renal failure but are often required for treatment of a variety of complications. Similarly, chronic renal failure patients present problems in surgical management of intercurrent illnesses. A high rate of infection and wound healing failures follow such surgical procedures. Preoperative dialysis, restoring all parameters of acid-base and electrolyte disequalibria, and lowering of the blood urea nitrogen and creatinine improve the risk considerably. Extensive drainage is routinely employed, and all wounds are managed with through-and-through closure techniques.

Peritoneal dialysis may be safely employed after laparotomy in these patients for 48 to 72 hours in most instances, even while spillage of visceral contents or bacterial peritonitis complicates its use. Appropriate antibiotics are added to the dialysis fluid, but in low doses, since the transperitoneal absorption of all antibiotics is virtually complete and excretion via the kidneys is very low.

The survival rate of postoperative patients with oliguric acute renal failure is only 55 per cent, despite close adherence to the rigid requirements of total care and dialysis outlined above.

REFERENCES

1. BAXTER, CR, ZEDLITZ, WH, AND SHIRES, GT: *High output acute renal failure complicating traumatic injury.* J Trauma 4:567, 1964.
2. SHIRES, GT, CARRICO, J, AND CANIZARO, PC: *Shock.* WB Saunders, Philadelphia, 1973, p 215.
3. BAXTER, CR, ET AL: *A practical method of renal hypothermia.* J Trauma 3:349, 1963.
4. STAHL, WM AND STONE, AM: *Effect of ethacrynic acid and furosemide on renal function in hypovolemia.* Ann Surg 174:1, 1971.
5. POWERS, SR: *Renal response to systematic trauma.* Am J Surg 199:603, 1970.
6. CRANDELL, SB, PAPPAS, SG, AND MACDONALD, A: *Nephrotoxicity associated with methoxyflurane anesthesia.* Anesthesiology 27:591, 1966.
7. BAKER, CR AND SHIRES, GT: *The evaluation of renal function following severe trauma.* J Trauma (in press).
8. FLEAR, CTG AND CLARKE, R: *The influence of blood loss and blood transfusion upon changes in the metabolism of water, electrolytes and nitrogen following civilian trauma.* Clin Sci 14:575, 1959.
9. BAXTER, CR AND MAYNARD, DR: *Prevention and recognition of surgical renal complications.* JENKINS, MP (ED): *Common and Uncommon Problems in Anesthesia,* Clinical Anesthesia Series, Vol 3. FA Davis, Philadelphia, 1968, p 321.
10. GRABER, IG AND SEVITT, S: *Renal function in burned patients and its relationship to morphological changes.* J Clin Path 12:25, 1959.
11. KUMIN, CM AND FINLAND, M: *Restrictions imposed on antibiotic therapy by renal failure.* Arch Intern Med 104:1030, 1959.
12. POWERS, SR: *Maintenance of renal function following massive trauma.* Trauma 10:554, 1970.

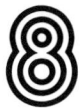

RATIONALE FOR BLOOD COMPONENT THERAPY

Karen Steinbronn, M.D., and
Douglas W. Huestis, M.D.

Doctors Steinbronn and Huestis are pathologists in charge of blood banking services at the University of Arizona Hospitals. Both are avid proponents of component therapy and represent majority opinion on this issue today. They offer several perspicuous statements concerning the advantages of component therapy. Among their salient points, the primary one is that use of component therapy allows wider utilization of blood and blood products. This is critically important in this era, when use of this scarce natural product is so widespread. Use of packed red cells ostensibly reduces the incidence of minor transfusion reactions, many of which have been ascribed to polymorphonuclear cells. An interesting fact brought out by these authors is that fewer microaggregates are found in packed red blood cells than in whole blood. The issue of fine versus coarse filtration for blood remains unresolved, but here is a feature of component therapy which clearly reduces the dimensions of the problem.

Although the authors describe the phenomenon of acute acidosis produced by massive blood transfusions secondary to acid citrate, they do not mention the aftermath. The anesthesiologist must be aware that the metabolic fallout at the conclusion of surgery requiring great numbers of transfusions may differ in each case. One mole of citrate (and one mole of lactate, for that matter) is metabolized to several moles of bicarbonate once effective liver perfusion and function are restored. This means that several hours following successful resuscitation, the patient may exhibit a paradoxical metabolic alkalosis. The practicing anesthesiologist will gain much insight from this chapter concerning the platelet washout phenomenon, various components derived from whole blood, and component utilization.

Burnell R. Brown, Jr.

The wide availability of blood products due to technologic advances has dramatically changed the practice of blood transfusion. Separation of freshly collected whole blood into multiple components is now accomplished in a closed system with the use of plastic bags, thus excluding bacterial contamination during preparation. Preservation requirements differ for the various blood constituents, and separation of whole blood into components allows for varied storage conditions and better preservation, concentration, and utilization of these precious human resources. Component therapy has largely replaced the use of whole blood in most parts of the country by offering specific products to replace specific deficits, although some circumstances still exist when whole blood may be the best product to transfuse if it is available. This article discusses the indications for and appropriate use of blood components and whole blood for the patient undergoing a surgical procedure (Table 1).

PREOPERATIVE BLOOD TRANSFUSION

Correction of anemia, the primary indication for transfusion of red blood cells, is ideally accomplished by the patient with the aid of appropriate specific therapy such as iron, folate, or vitamin B_{12}. If the cause of the anemia is iron deficiency, adequate iron therapy should result in reticulocytosis peaking within 7 to 10 days of treatment, a significant hemoglobin rise in three to four weeks, and a normal hemoglobin value in two months.[1] Often neither the surgeon nor the patient is willing to delay a surgical procedure to this extent, and preoperative blood transfusion may then be considered desirable.

In general, preoperative transfusion has been considered unnecessary if the patient's hematocrit is above 30 percent, corresponding to a hemoglobin level above 10 g per dl, and if the patient's cardiac, pulmonary, hepatic and renal functions are normal.[2] This number is based primarily on data from animal studies showing a depression of ventricular function when the hemoglobin level falls below 10 g per dl in acute dilutional anemia.[3] With further hemodilution, compensatory mechanisms such as coronary vasodilation and increased heart rate can no longer compensate for the anemia, and myocardial hypoxia is likely. Other studies have shown that the increased coronary flow of acute anemia was sufficient to maintain a normal coronary sinus oxygen tension even with a hematocrit of 20 percent, but this level is not considered adequate for elective surgery.[4] In each case, the patient's cardiac status must be considered, as well as the type of surgery and possibility of operative blood loss. The expected benefits of preoperative transfusion must outweigh the known hazards of transfusion. Reactions to blood transfusion are common, and generally reported in about 6 to 7 percent of patients transfused.[5] Most reactions are minor, such as allergic or febrile, nonhemolytic reactions; but there is an ever-present risk of serious hemolytic reaction. In the series of Baker, Moinichen, and Nyhus,[6] hemolytic reactions occurred in 35 of 42,331 recipients, and eight of these patients died. Besides these immediate reactions, there is also a risk of delayed complications such as viral hepatitis.

Transfusion of each unit of red blood cells in a 70 kg patient should raise the hematocrit by 3 percentage points, corresponding to a hemoglobin rise of 1 g per dl, and the amount needed for a particular patient can easily be determined.[7] In an adult, transfusion of a single unit of red blood cells is usually considered to be of little or no benefit, since a change of 3 percentage points is of minimal clinical significance. If the anemia is severe enough to require transfusion for improved oxygenation, at least 2 units of red blood cells are usually necessary.

When possible, preoperative blood transfusion should take place 24 hours before surgery for several reasons. Some of the storage defects of banked red blood cells will be reversed in that period. During storage there is a decrease in red cell adenosine triphosphate (ATP), which is associated with a change in the red cell shape from a biconcave disk to a sphere with an increase in cellular rigidity. Stored cells also lose 2,3-diphosphoglycerate (2,3-DPG) causing an increased affinity of hemoglobin for oxygen. When stored cells depleted of 2,3-DPG are transfused, the level returns to 50 percent of normal within 24 hours, becoming normal by 48 hours.[8] This storage defect probably becomes important only in those patients receiving large volumes of banked blood. During storage, potassium leaks out of the red cells and sodium enters. The transfused cells will regain their normal electrolyte concentration in the recipient. It has been shown that a normal sodium content will be restored within 24 hours, although potassium restoration takes longer.[8] Following transfusion, increased blood in the pulmonary vasculature may alter pulmonary function until the blood volume has had time to equilibrate.[2]

Finally, a preoperative evaluation of hemostasis must be included to anticipate special operative blood needs of the patient and to identify any bleeding problems. A careful history of bleeding tendencies and the use of drugs affecting hemostasis is the most important part of the evaluation. If a major surgical procedure is planned, and

Table 1. Blood components

Name	Volume	Contents	Clinical uses
Red Blood Cells	300 ml	Red cells. Some plasma, leukocytes and platelets.	Anemia. Blood loss.
Whole Blood	500 ml	Red cells, plasma, leukocytes and platelets.	Massive blood loss.
Frozen Red Blood Cells	200–250 ml	Red cells. No plasma. Almost no leukocytes or platelets.	Anemia. Storage of rare bloods. Patients who may not receive donor protein or leukocytes.
Red Blood Cells, Leukocyte Poor	200–250 ml	Red cells. Some plasma. Few leukocytes. Few platelets.	Anemia. Patients who may not receive donor leukocytes.
Platelets (conventional)	30–50 ml	Platelets. Lymphocytes. Some plasma.	Bleeding due to thrombocytopenia or thrombocytopathy.

Platelets (by cytapheresis)	200–400 ml	Platelets. Variable lymphocytes and plasma.	As above, for patients refractory to regular platelets.
Leukocytes	200–600 ml	Leukocytes, variable. Platelets. Some red blood cells.	Neutropenia and infection.
Fresh Frozen Plasma	200 ml	Plasma. All coagulation factors.	Provide clotting factors. Hemophilia B.
Cryoprecipitate	10–25 ml	Factors I and VIII. Some plasma.	Hemophilia A. Von Willebrands Disease. Fibrinogen deficiency.

depending on the clinical background, baseline laboratory tests, including a prothrombin time, partial thromboplastin time, and platelet count may be advisable. Of course, a history of bleeding problems requires definitive investigation. The management of patients with coagulopathies will be discussed in a later section.

For many surgical procedures, blood is routinely crossmatched as a precautionary measure, but is rarely transfused. Recently, it has been recommended that each hospital study its own blood use patterns.[9,10] For procedures in which the average number of units transfused per case is half a unit or less, ABO and Rh typing and an antibody screen on the patient's serum are recommended, rather than a type and crossmatch, provided that appropriate blood units are available and the antibody screen is negative. The use of the type and screen allows for discovery of unexpected antibodies and identifies patients for whom compatible blood may be difficult to find. These problems can be solved in advance of surgery at no increased risk to the patient. The type and antibody screen has been shown to be 99.99 percent effective in preventing the transfusion of incompatible blood.[11] At the same time, the type and antibody screen eliminates unnecessary crossmatches and the practice of reserving particular units for a particular patient in a situation where the patient is not likely to receive any blood. When a unit is crossmatched, it must be removed from general use and placed on reserve, usually for 24 to 48 hours. When such a unit is not transfused, its available shelf life is reduced, increasing its likelihood of outdating. If, during a procedure, the patient who has been typed and screened requires blood, type-specific units can immediately be dispatched, and the crossmatch readily done. This practice decreases blood bank workload, reduces cost, allows for reduced inventories of blood, and has been shown to be safe for the patient.

USE OF WHOLE BLOOD

The current trend in blood transfusion is to component therapy and the treatment of a specific deficit with a specific blood product. Thus, whole blood has become less available, and often is unavailable on short notice. A unit of whole blood has a volume of approximately 500 ml and contains red cells, plasma, leukocytes, platelets, and clotting factors mixed with an anticoagulant solution. These are in various concentrations and states of preservation, depending on the duration of storage and other variables. Whole blood usually does not supply adequate platelets or labile clotting factors unless it is very fresh, and none of its constituents is in a concentrated state. Platelets in whole blood, for example, are no longer useful after 24 hours of storage.[12] Factors V and VIII are the most labile of the clotting factors, and have less than 50 percent activity after one week of storage.[13] In cases of significant blood loss, when both plasma and red cells are required, whole blood can satisfy the need. Usually, clinical situations of massive blood loss are not foreseen, and whole blood may not be readily available. Although stored whole blood can supply red cells as well as volume, significant blood loss can also be adequately treated by appropriate components. Whole blood should not be used in the belief that it represents what the patient lost, since once stored, its various constituents become altered. In addition, it has foreign antigens and accumulated metabolites.

For the correction of anemia and moderate blood loss, transfusion of red blood cells should be the rule. Among the disadvantages of red cells are slow flow rate, inadequate volume replacement in acute blood loss, and lower amount of plasma protein and coagulation factors. The flow rate of red blood cells can be improved by dilution with normal saline, thus achieving a rapid rate. Although red blood cells alone may be inadequate in supplying volume in massive acute hemorrhage, the concurrent use of plasma volume expanders and other components will adequately treat hypovolemia. The small amount of protein in whole blood is insignificant nutritionally. Finally, the deficiency of labile coagulation factors becomes important only in massive transfusion, and as noted above, also exists in whole blood.

The advantage of red blood cells over whole blood is decreased volume load. The hematocrit of a unit of red blood cells is 70 percent, compared with 30 to 40 percent in a unit of whole blood. A smaller volume can be given to achieve the same increase in oxygen-carrying capacity, which may be essential in patients with congestive heart failure or others in danger of fluid overload. The removal of plasma decreases the total amount of electrolytes and citrate in the unit of red cells. The reduction of sodium and protein may be beneficial to certain cardiac patients.

The major advantage of red blood cells over whole blood is the economic utilization of blood as a resource. The demands to supply platelets, plasma, and cryoprecipitate for specific patients, and the fact that the majority of transfusions are to correct anemia, has led blood banks to favor the production of components. Components such as platelets and antihemophilic factor can then be concentrated and stored under optimal conditions.

TRANSFUSION DURING SURGERY

In most surgical procedures blood loss is minimal, less than 1000 ml, or below 20 percent of the adult patient's blood volume. Blood volume is variable and related to the individual's body size and sex, and can easily be determined from appropriate formulas or nomograms, such as those given by the American Association of Blood Banks.[14] For each patient, blood volume should be estimated before surgery to allow proper evaluation of fluid losses. The anesthesiologist aims to maintain the patient's full blood volume. Plasma substitutes alone are currently used when blood losses are not so great as to necessitate blood transfusion to maintain an adequate hematocrit.

The use of either crystalloid or colloid solutions causes hemodilution. This may not be tolerated by patients with pre-existing cardiovascular or pulmonary disease, although those with adequate cardiac status can compensate for the decreased hematocrit with increased cardiac output. Patients who have a lowered hematocrit at the start may not tolerate further hemodilution without red cell replacement.

An important aspect of hemodilution is the decrease in blood viscosity that allows for increased peripheral flow.[15] This, together with increased cardiac output, causes increased total blood flow to most organs. The reduction in blood viscosity is transient when crystalloids are infused because of the rapid loss of fluid into the extravascular space. Fluid overload may result from the attempt to maintain the blood volume with crystalloids, and postoperative diuretics may be necessary. On the other hand, the decrease in viscosity effected by colloid solutions is more stable because the increased oncotic pressure maintains the blood volume. Dextran 40 decreases the blood viscosity out of proportion to the drop in hematocrit, decreases platelet adhesiveness, thus prolonging bleeding time, and alters the structure of fibrin, causing increased fibrinolysis.[16] There are reports of reduced incidence of postoperative pulmonary emboli in patients receiving dextran either intraoperatively or early in the postoperative period.[17] If dextran is used, it usually causes laboratory difficulty in typing and crossmatching blood, so samples for crossmatching must be drawn before infusion of dextran, if at all possible.

Operative blood loss *above* 20 percent of the patient's blood volume lowers the hematocrit to the range of 30 to 35 percent, and usually necessitates blood transfusion. Even in patients who have adapted to a chronic anemia, a sudden drop such as that with acute blood loss is poorly tolerated. Again, the generalization holds, that if blood transfusion is necessary to improve oxygenation, at least 2 units of red cells be given (in adults), since lesser amounts seldom produce a significant clinical effect, and may needlessly expose the patient to the risks of transfusion. Each unit of red blood cells has a volume of about 300 ml to be calculated into the fluid input.

Banked red cells should be exposed only to isotonic saline during transfusion. If given in a hypotonic solution such as half- or quarter-strength saline, direct hemolysis will take place. The use of dextrose solutions to suspend red cells causes swelling of the cells and decreased survival time.[18] Ringer's lactate solution contains ionized calcium and may cause clotting.

The standard transfusion filter is a 170-μm filter; however, stored blood contains microaggregates of platelets, fibrin strands, and cellular debris which are small enough to pass through the standard filter. These can be eliminated by microfilters with a pore size of 25- to 40-μm. It is standard procedure in many operating rooms to use microaggregate filters for all blood transfusions, although patients receiving moderate amounts of stored blood appear to be able to handle the transfused microaggregates without side effects. Since microaggregates develop and increase mostly after the first week of storage, the age and the quantity of blood are important factors in deciding whether significant amounts of microaggregates are present.[19] Most studies of microaggregate formation have included analysis of whole blood only; however, Gervin and associates[20] have shown that the majority of microaggregates form from the leukocytes and platelets of the buffy coat, and few microaggregates are present in concentrated red blood cells.

Microemboli have been demonstrated in the lungs of patients given large volumes of stored blood, and there is some evidence to suggest that these emboli may have clinically significant effects on pulmonary function.[21] In one study, 16 patients each received more than 1000 ml of stored blood during surgery, and had normal pulmonary function before surgery. In eight of these patients, standard transfusion filters alone were used, and this group had significantly higher ventilation-to-perfusion ratios and increased arterial blood pH when compared with the eight patients who received blood transfused through microaggregate filters. Another group has reported an increase in pulmonary arteriovenous (A-V) shunting and a decrease in the diffusion capacity when patients received more than 20 percent of their blood volume through standard filters.[22] Unfortunately, in these studies, the patients were few and the variables many. Furthermore, clinical studies in humans and animals have looked mainly at the effects of microaggregates in the transfusion of whole blood, and studies documenting effects of microaggregates in red blood cell transfusions are lacking. Microaggregate filters may have a place in the transfusion of large volumes of older stored blood, although not all authorities agree with this. Several microaggregate filters are currently available commercially, and a recent study compares their effectiveness and flow rates.[23]

Blood warmers are frequently used for intraoperative transfusion, but are of importance only in the rapid transfusion of large amounts of cold stored blood. The combination of rapid transfusion of chilled blood, a cool operating room, and exposed body cavities and viscera may cause significant hypothermia. Hypothermia may contribute to decreased organ perfusion, hypoxia, acidosis, and cardiac arrhythmia. When the body temperature drops below 32°C, there is a risk of ventricular fibrillation. The risk of hypothermia is minimal at the usual transfusion rates. Blood warmers must be monitored, since overheating can cause hemolysis.

MASSIVE TRANSFUSION

Transfusion of large amounts of banked blood may be required during major surgery or trauma, and as transfusion continues, the patient's blood starts to resemble banked blood, and hemostasis is altered. Initially, the mixture of transfused blood and the patient's own blood contains sufficient coagulation factors, but with continued blood loss and utilization of clotting factors, these factors may become depleted. The amount of transfused blood necessary to cause defective hemostasis varies in each patient, but is usually more than 20 units of red blood cells. Above this amount, a unit of fresh frozen plasma can be given for each 4 units of red cells to replenish coagulation factors.

Although a reserve of platelets can be released from the bone marrow in situations of stress, massive transfusion of blood will have a dilutional effect on the circulating level of platelets. Again, this effect is most likely to become significant following the transfusion of 20 or so units of red blood cells. The platelet count will usually drop to approximately 50,000 per μl regardless of the pretransfusion platelet level. This level is usually adequate to prevent spontaneous bleeding, but may be inadequate to control hemorrhage in a patient already bleeding. A sufficient dose of platelets should be given, normally not less than 4×10^{11} platelets to an adult, corresponding to 6 to 8 platelet concentrates.[24]

Banked blood contains citrate as part of the anticoagulant solution, and massive transfusions therefore include excess citrate. Citrate is rapidly metabolized by the body, and unless the patient has liver failure or reduced organ perfusion, toxic levels of citrate are very unlikely. Signs of citrate toxicity are likely only in rapid transfusion, when blood is given at a rate greater than 1 unit per 5 minutes in an adult.[25] The hazard of citrate toxicity is related to hypocalcemia, which may occur when citrate binds calcium in the recipient. Muscle tremors and prolongation of the QT interval in the electrocardiogram may occur due to hypocalcemia. These changes can be reversed with the administration of calcium gluconate or calcium chloride. The routine use of calcium during massive transfusion is controversial, since hypocalcemia is often difficult to document, and the administration of calcium can be dangerous. Wolf, McCarthy, and Hafleigh[26] reported a fatal cardiac arrest associated with hypercalcemia in a child following transfusions combined with calcium administration. The use of the calcium ion-sensitive electrode for the measurement of ionized calcium has allowed accurate quantification of the calcium level that may have been lacking in older reports of citrate toxicity with hypocalcemia. Recent studies indicate that it is rarely necessary to administer calcium to improve cardiac function, except during special procedures such as open heart surgery.[27,28]

An acid-base imbalance can occur with rapid massive blood transfusion. This is primarily due to the citric acid and lactic acid of stored blood. The problem of acidosis is diminished with the anticoagulant citrate-phosphate-dextrose (CPD), since CPD has a higher pH than acid-citrate-dextrose (ACD). In previously healthy subjects, the base deficiency is rapidly corrected.[29] However, some recommend correction of the acidosis by exogenous methods, such as the administration of 50 mEq of sodium bicarbonate for every 5 units of blood given.[30]

Potassium toxicity has been considered a problem of massive transfusion because of the elevated plasma levels of potassium in stored blood. As red blood cells are stored, potassium leaks from the cell and sodium enters. The concentration of plasma potassium in a unit of CPDA-1 red blood cells at 35 days of storage at 4°C is in the range of 70 mEq per liter; but since a unit of red blood cells contains less than 100 ml of plasma, it would require at least 10 units to give 70 mEq of potassium. Once the red cells are transfused, they restore their normal electrolyte concentration, thus hypokalemia may be seen after massive transfusion of older stored blood.

The current standard methods of storing blood are associated with a loss of 2,3-DPG from the red cells after a variable period. This increases the affinity of hemoglobin for oxygen, so that hemoglobin in stored blood becomes less efficient for delivering oxygen at physiologic gas tensions. Because the normal levels of 2,3-DPG are restored rapidly in the recipient, it is not a problem in the majority of transfused patients. However, there has been considerable interest in the effects of diminished 2,3-DPG in massive transfusions, although so far the data have been contradictory. The majority of studies show no deleterious effects, probably because alterations of oxygen affinity can be compensated for by increased cardiac output, increased blood flow to tissues, and capillary dilatation.[25,31,32] Others believe the level of 2,3-DPG is important in patients with marginal cardiac reserve. In one study of patients undergoing coronary artery bypass surgery, those transfused with blood having decreased levels of 2,3-DPG were shown to have a decreased cardiac index compared with patients transfused with blood having elevated levels of 2,3-DPG.[33] In this study, there were many other variables that could not be controlled. The levels of 2,3-DPG are well maintained in blood stored in CPD up to a week. Patients with altered cardiac status receiving large volumes of banked blood should probably receive blood less than one week old to avoid the possibility of detrimental cardiac effects.

Other problems associated with massive transfusion include hypothermia and microembolization, discussed above.

SURGICAL BLEEDING

Most often, bleeding in the surgical patient is mechanical, a result of interrupted vascular spaces which can be controlled by surgical hemostasis. This type of bleeding is localized, in contrast to the usually generalized bleeding associated with a defect in the coagulation mechanism.

Excessive bleeding noted when a skin incision is made is usually due to a deficiency in platelet numbers or function, excessive anticoagulation, or an unexpected coagulation factor deficiency. The procedure should be delayed while appropriate coagulation tests are done to identify the problem.

Unexpected bleeding during surgery may be caused by a deficiency of platelets or coagulation factors, consumptive coagulopathy, or hyperfibrinolysis. If there has been administration of large volumes of banked blood without replacement of platelets or coagulation factors, the bleeding may be solely due to this dilutional effect. Laboratory studies must be done to determine the cause of the bleeding problem and the appropriate treatment.

Useful tests during active bleeding include a platelet count, prothrombin time (PT), partial thromboplastin time (PTT), fibrinogen concentration, and concentration of fibrin degradation products. If the patient has a known clotting factor deficiency, that factor concentration should be assayed.

If the platelet count is abnormally low (less than 50,000) with normal PT and PTT values, bleeding is probably due to thromobocytopenia, and platelet concentrates should be given. In the event that the platelet count is normal, but either the PT or PTT is prolonged, fresh frozen plasma can be administered to provide coagulation factors.

In consumptive coagulopathy, such as disseminated intravascular coagulation (DIC), both platelets and coagulation factors are consumed. The patient has a low platelet count, usually less than that seen with dilutional thrombocytopenia. The PT and PTT are prolonged and the fibrinogen concentration is below 150 mg per dl. Furthermore, in DIC, the level of fibrin degradation products is greater than 40 mcg per ml. The administration of fresh frozen plasma, cryoprecipitate, or platelets may fail to correct the hemostasis, and may even feed the consumptive coagulopathy. Intraoperatively, DIC is often due to tumor, aneurysm, abscess, or a dead fetus; and unless the cause can be removed in a short time, the coagulopathy should be slowed with heparin before giving platelets or cryoprecipitate. Heparin is not usually used during surgery because it may increase bleeding; however, in some instances it may be necessary. The average adult patient should receive 2500 to 4000 units as a loading dose, and 800 to 1000 units per hour as a constant infusion until the cause of the DIC can be corrected.[34] In cases of abnormal surgical bleeding, communication with the blood bank physician can be invaluable in selecting the appropriate laboratory tests and corrective therapy for the patient.

The patient with liver disease presents a special problem, since the defect in hemostasis can have many causes. The vitamin K dependent factors II, VII, IX and X that are synthesized in the liver are frequently diminished. This problem can be alleviated by administering fresh frozen plasma to supply these factors, and monitoring the prothrombin time. These patients frequently have splenomegaly on the basis of portal hypertension, resulting in sequestration of platelets, and thrombocytopenia. Usually the thrombocytopenia is only moderate, and the patient has a normal bleeding time. However, with hemorrhage and red cell transfusion, such patients may develop further thrombocytopenia on the basis of dilution, and may require platelet concentrates for hemostasis. Thus, the platelet count should also be monitored.

Cardiac surgery with cardiopulmonary bypass produces alterations in hemostasis that are not fully understood. Thrombocytopenia has been reported by many investigators, and some have shown the decrease in platelets to be related to the pump time, while others have found no relationship. The most commonly cited explanations for thrombocytopenia include: a dilutional effect owing to the nonblood prime in the oxygenator apparatus, platelet utilization in the pump, or disseminated intravascular coagulation.[35] Defects in platelet function have also been reported.[36,37] Salzman[38] showed decreased platelet adhesiveness on glass beads after bypass. More recently, Harker and associates[39] have attributed the platelet dysfunction to a selective alpha granule release from platelets during bypass. Patients who have come off cardiopulmonary bypass may have abnormal bleeding with a prolonged bleeding time (greater than 20 minutes), in spite of platelet counts above 100,000 μl. Such patients have been shown to benefit from the transfusion of platelet concentrates.

Various coagulation factor deficiencies have been reported under such circumstances, although hypofibrinogenemia has been noted most frequently. Bick[35] has suggested that primary hyperfibrinolysis is a more likely cause of hypofibrinogenemia than disseminated intravascular coagulation because of heparinization and frequently minimal thrombocytopenia. Plasmin levels are usually elevated from the activation of plasminogen during bypass. There is usually improvement in hemostasis after bypass, and the reversal of heparin with protamine sulfate. Replacement therapy with fresh frozen plasma, cryoprecipitate, and platelets is usually effective. Rarely, the fibrinolysis may become so brisk as to warrant the use of epsilon aminocaproic acid as an inhibitor of fibrinolysis.

CONCLUSION

Routine separation of blood into components has become the standard procedure in blood banks, resulting in more economic utilization of this resource. Specific products are now provided to replace specific deficits, without exposing the patient to unnecessary substances that could also be harmful to certain individuals. Blood transfusion has become more complex with component therapy, in that many products are now available. Transfusion of blood components during surgery is now usual, and although not all clinical settings could be discussed in this article, the anesthesiologist needs to be aware of the composition of various components of blood and the circumstances in which each is used.

REFERENCES

1. FAIRBANKS, VF AND BEUTLER, E: *Iron deficiency.* In WILLIAMS, WJ (ED): Hematology, ed 2. McGraw-Hill, New York, 1977, p 376.
2. MOLLISON, PL: *Blood Transfusion in Clinical Medicine,* ed. 6. Blackwell Scientific Publications, Oxford, 1979,
3. CASE, RB, BERGLUND, E, AND SARNOFF, SJ: *Ventricular function: Changes in coronary resistance and ventricular function resulting from acute induced anemia and the effect thereon of coronary stenosis.* Am J Med 18:397, 1955.
4. MURRAY, JF AND RAPAPORT, E: *Myocardial metabolism in acute normovolemic anemia.* Clin Res 16:144, 1968.
5. HUESTIS, DW: *Acute transfusion reaction.* In CONN, HF and CONN, II, RB (eds): Current Diagnosis 6. WB Saunders, Philadelphia, 1980, p 459.
6. BAKER, RJ, MOINICHEN, SL, and NYHUS, LM: *Transfusion reaction: A reappraisal of surgical incidence and significance.* Ann Surg 169:684, 1969.
7. WIDMAN, FK (ED) American Association of Blood Banks Technical manual, JB Lippincott, Philadelphia, 1981, p 263.
8. VALERI, CR AND HIRSCH, NM: *Restoration of in vivo erythrocyte adenosine triphosphate, 2,3-diphosphoglycerate, potassium ion, and sodium ion concentration following transfusion of acid-citrate-dextrose stored human red blood cells.* J Lab Clin Med 73:722, 1969.
9. SARMA, DP: *Use of blood in elective surgery.* JAMA 243:1536, 1980.
10. BORAL, LI, DANNEMILLER, FJ, AND STANFORD, W, ET AL: *A guideline for anticipated blood usage during elective surgical procedures.* Am J Clin Pathol 71:680, 1979.
11. BORAL, LI, AND HENRY, JB: *The type and screen: A safe alternative and supplement in selected surgical procedures.* Transfusion 17:165, 1977.
12. BALDINI, M, COSTEA, N, AND DAMESHEK, W: *The viability of stored human platelets.* Blood 16:1669, 1960.
13. RAPAPORT, SI, AMES, SB, AND MIKKELSEN, S: *The levels of antihemophilic globulin and proaccelerin in fresh and bank blood.* Am J Clin Pathol 31:297, 1959.
14. AMERICAN ASSOCIATION OF BLOOD BANKS: *Blood Component Therapy. A Physician's Handbook.* AABB, Washington, DC, 1975, p 7.

15. MESSMER, K: *Hemodilution.* Surg Clin North Am 55:659, 1975.
16. BERGENTZ, SE: *On bleeding and clotting problems in post-traumatic states.* Crit Care Med 4:41, 1976.
17. HARRIS, WH, ET AL: *Prevention of venous thromboembolism following total hip replacement.* JAMA 220:1319, 1972.
18. RYDEN, SE AND OBERMAN, HA: *Compatibility of common intravenous solutions with CPD blood.* Transfusion 15:250, 1975.
19. SOLIS, RT, ET AL: *Physical characteristics of microaggregates in stored blood.* Transfusion 14:538, 1974.
20. GERVIN, A, et al: *Source of microaggregates in stored human blood.* Clin Res 22:177, 1974.
21. TAKAORI, M, NAKAJO, N, AND ISHII, T: *Changes of pulmonary function following transfusion of stored blood.* Transfusion 17:615, 1977.
22. BARRETT, J, TAHIR, AH, AND LITWIN, MS: *Increased pulmonary arteriovenous shunting in humans following blood transfusion.* Arch Surg 113:947, 1978.
23. CULLEN, DJ, ET AL: *Comparative evaluation of new fine-screen filters: Effects on blood flow rate and microaggregate removal.* Anesthesiology 53:3, 1980.
24. INTERNATIONAL SOCIETY OF BLOOD TRANSFUSION: *Blood Component Therapy.* International Society of Blood Transfusion, Paris, 1980.
25. COLLINS, JA: *Problems associated with the massive transfusion of stored blood.* Surgery 75:274, 1974.
26. WOLF, PL, MCCARTHY, LJ, AND HAFLEIGH, B: *Extreme hypercalcemia following blood transfusion combined with intravenous calcium.* Vox Sang 19:544, 1970.
27. HOWLAND, WS, et al: *The cardiovascular effects of low levels of ionized calcium during massive transfusion.* Surg Gynecol Obstet 145:581, 1977.
28. PERKINS, HA, et al: *Calcium ion activity during rapid exchange transfusion with citrated blood.* Transfusion 11:204, 1971.
29. COLLINS, JA, ET AL: *Acid-base status of seriously wounded combat casualties II. Resuscitation with stored blood.* Ann Surg 173:6, 1971.
30. *Massive transfusion.* In GREENWALT, TJ (ED): *General Principles of Blood Transfusion.* American Medical Association, Chicago, 1977, p 13.
31. WRANNE, B, NORDGREN, L, AND WOODSON, RD: *Increased blood oxygen affinity and physical work capacity in man.* Scand J Clin Lab Invest 33:347, 1974.
32. LICHTMAN, MA, ET AL: *The relationships between arterial oxygen flow rate, oxygen binding by hemoglobin and oxygen utilization after myocardial infarction.* J Clin Invest 54:501, 1974.

33. DENNIS, RC, ET AL: *Improved myocardial performance following high 2,3-DPG red cell transfusion.* Surgery 77:741, 1975.
34. SILVER, D AND HARRINGTON, MP: *Disorderly hemostasis.* In CONDON, RE AND DE CASSE, JJ (EDS): *Surgical Care.* Lea & Febiger, Philadelphia, 1980, p 173.
35. BICK, RL: *Alterations of hemostasis associated with cardiopulmonary bypass: Pathophysiology, prevention, diagnosis and management.* Seminars in Thrombosis and Hemostasis 3(2):59, 1976.
36. MCKENNA, R, ET AL: *The hemostatic mechanism after open-heart surgery II: Frequency of abnormal platelet function during and after extracorporeal circulation.* J Thorac Cardiovasc Surg 70:298, 1975.
37. KALTER, RD, ET AL: *Cardiopulmonary bypass associated hemostatic abnormalities.* J Thorac Cardiovasc Surg 77:427, 1979.
38. SALZMAN, WE: *Blood platelets and extracorporeal circulation.* Transfusion 3:274, 1963.
39. HARKER, LA, ET AL: *Mechanism of abnormal bleeding in patients undergoing cardiopulmonary bypass.* Blood 56:824, 1980.

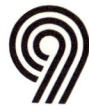

PRACTICAL CONSIDERATIONS IN TRANSFUSION TECHNIQUES DURING ANESTHESIA

Reynolds J. Saunders, M.D., and
Jerry M. Calkins, M.D., Ph.D.

Engineers to the rescue! The problems related to blood transfusion and component therapy are not all biochemical or physiologic. Just getting packed red blood cells to flow at a rate commensurate with need is at times sufficient impediment to destroy all theoretic considerations of the advantages of component therapy. To make matters worse, when component therapy was first introduced, I am not embarrassed to admit that I diluted the first few units of red cells I administered with Ringer's lactate! This is now known to be anathema, as there is sufficient calcium in Hartmann's solution to bind the anticoagulant citrate.

Dr. Saunders and Calkins from the Bioengineering Research Section of Anesthesiology at the College of Medicine, University of Arizona, review the rheologic and viscosity problems inherent in blood transfusions. Red cell stresses and shears and implications are discussed. Pragmatic considerations referable to various intravenous tubing connections are covered. An issue not covered at length is concern over the advantages and disadvantages of micropore filters. Are they overrated? Enthusiasm for these devices has ranged from unanimous heuristic acceptance to mordant rejection. In truth, there has never been unequivocal documentation that micropore filters reduce mortality and morbidity, even during massive transfusions. This is a curious phenomenon, since use of these rather expensive devices is widespread. It is hoped that data may be collected in the future which will help resolve the problem. Until that time, the admonition of "clinical judgment" holds.

Burnell R. Brown, Jr.

The folklore related to transfusion technique is precariously rooted in misinformation, misunderstanding, and misapplication. Although a great deal is known about the chemical and physical changes in blood that result from various techniques of storage, the practicing anesthesiologist often must rely on scanty data and intuition for guidance in transfusion techniques for surgery. Nevertheless, enough information is now available so that a review of current techniques in transfusion therapy may be of value, to both the anesthesiologist and the patient. Because we deal with a perishable commodity that is collected, prepared, and stored outside our supervision or control, our task must be to insure that blood and components arrive in the patient's bloodstream with the highest possible state of function. Since the damage incurred before we receive these products is rarely reversible, it is crucial to avoid further impairment or destruction when they are administered.

This chapter explores factors affecting acceptable transfusion techniques (Fig. 1). Biochemical factors affecting blood products will be ignored (in spite of their great importance), since these factors are largely beyond the control of the anesthesiologist during surgery. The physical stresses which alter the composition or function of blood products (Fig. 2), and the equipment which produces these stresses are covered, followed by a description of individual components and their susceptibility to various stresses. Some precautions which prudence dictates are considered, and some hazards, both obvious and obscure, are discussed. Many recommendations are supported by research, and the rest may be ascribed to standard procedures in the authors' Department of Anesthesiology.

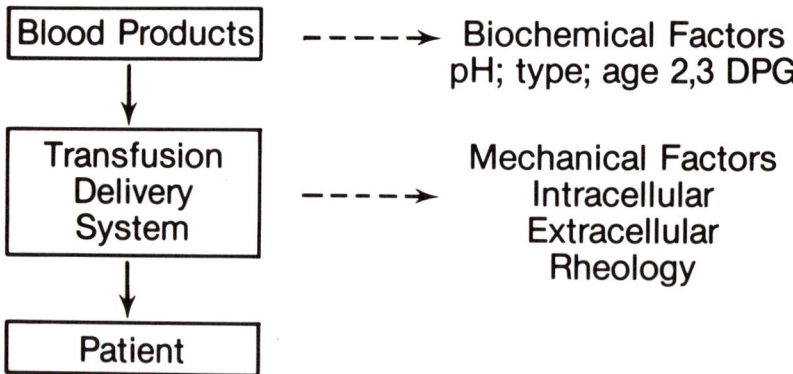

Figure 1. Factors affecting component viability.

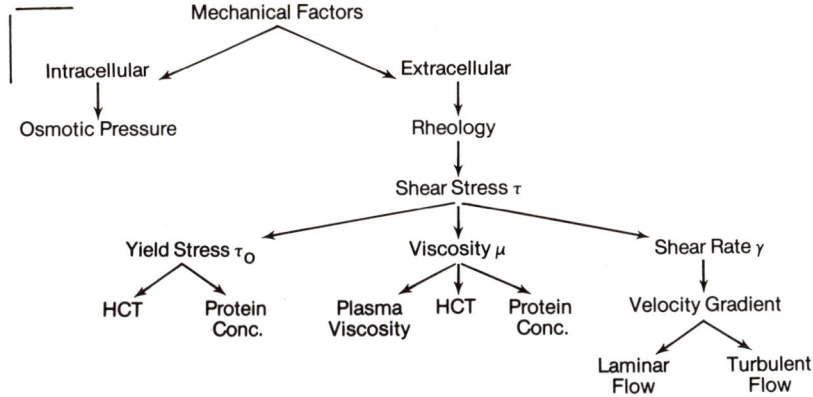

Figure 2. Transfusion delivery system.

PHYSICAL FACTORS

Anesthesiologists have some degree of control over the physical environment to which blood products are subjected after storage and before entrance into the patient's bloodstream. We will consider the physical factors in the order in which they are ordinarily encountered in the operating room environment.

Osmotic Factors

Maintenance of the integrity and function of red blood cells and other cellular components of blood requires special care. When collected, these components are in an isotonic medium, the plasma. In a period of prolonged storage, the normal metabolism of the cellular components is slowed, and potassium and ammonium ions accumulate in the plasma. Valeri and Hirsch[1] have shown that red blood cells damaged by storage nevertheless can be restored in the recipient after: (1) 2,3-diphosphoglycerate (2,3-DPG) and adenosine triphosphate (ATP) levels are restored, (2) the potassium ion level is increased within the cells, and (3) the elevated carbon dioxide tension (P_{CO_2}) and nonexistent ionized calcium level present in the storage medium are returned to normal. Prior to that restoration, red blood cells and other cellular components must be regarded as being particularly susceptible to osmotic influences during transfer and infusion (Fig. 3).

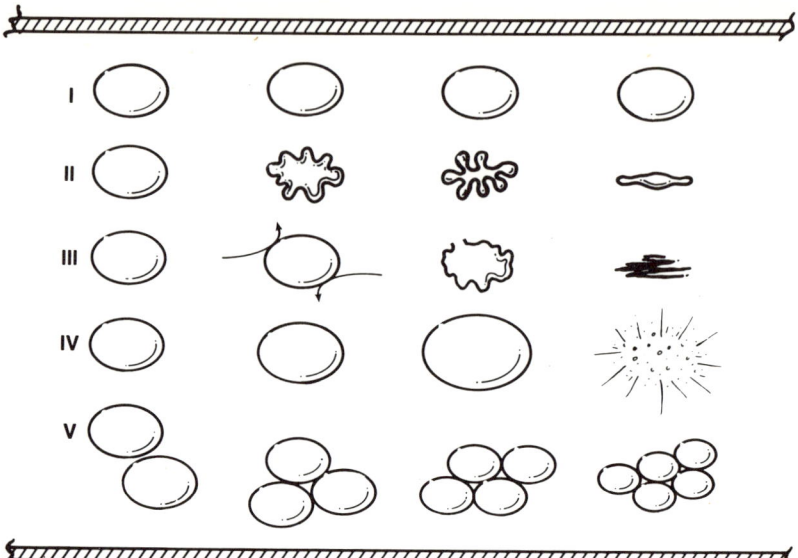

Figure 3. Factors affecting viability. (I) Nothing happens: solution, apparatus, flow normal. (II) Shrink: hypertonic solution. (III) Forces tear apart: mechanical factors. (IV) Swell, explode: hypotonic solution. (V) Aggregate, clump: biochemical factors.

Jones, Kilpatrick, and Franks[2] showed in human subjects that simply supplying an isotonic environment is not sufficient to protect red blood cells from damage. They demonstrated that exposure to the isotonic solution 5 percent dextrose caused crenation (shrinkage) and agglutination of red blood cells, which when resuspended in plasma changed into morphologically—if not functionally—normal forms. Nevertheless, up to 74 percent of the infused red blood cells were removed from the patient's circulation within 48 hours after administration. The authors explain the cause of this effect as the absence of electrolytes in the solution to which the cells are exposed, not the tonicity of the solution. As a result of exposure, the selective permeability of the cell membrane is changed so that chloride, bicarbonate, and potassium leave the cell. This exodus causes basic biochemical changes in cellular function which contribute to the shortened life expectancy.

Although varying hypertonic combinations of 5 percent dextrose and sodium chloride have been advocated for preservation of cells, the addition of salt does not prevent shortened cellular lifespan. No significant damage to cellular components has been demonstrated from use of 0.9 percent sodium chloride solution (isotonic normal saline) as a suspension medium.[2] Unfortunately, one continues to encounter colleagues who use dextrose-containing solutions for resuspension of red blood cells. Although correctly aware that agglutination of red blood cells per se is reversible, they are unaware that red cell survival may be drastically shortened by the process of agglutination. When a colloid solution is preferred to saline, we have found that fresh frozen plasma, because it is isotonic, may be used quite handily for suspension of red cells without apparent harm. In addition, all anesthesiologists should be aware of the danger of hemolysis which results from cell volume expansion due to utilization of hypotonic solutions (0.45 percent sodium chloride, 2.5 percent dextrose, and so forth), either for infusion or for suspension of blood components. Water injures the cell membrane and produces an increase in intracellular pressure, resulting in rupture of the cell.

Temperature Factors

Anesthesiologists have two main interests in warming blood products prior to infusion: the first is to avoid the danger of lowering total body temperature in an already poikilothermic patient; the second is the risk of massive transfusion through a central line, provoking arrhythmias or even cardiac arrest, due to the sudden infusion of cold liquid. Boyan[3] reported that cardiac arrests during massive transfusions were lowered from 58 to 7 percent by warming blood to body temperature before infusion. In addition, the increased viscosity due to low temperature leads to increased destruction of red blood cells during transfusion. It is essential to know the proper methods for warming blood products to avoid loss of activity of the components.

Within limits of 4 to 40°C, the short-term survival of blood components does not seem to be affected. Thus, at one moment the components may be stored at 4°C, and at the next moment they may be rapidly rewarmed to 37 to 40°C without apparent harm. Temperatures lower than 4°C or higher than 40°C are likely to cause hemolysis or denaturation of plasma proteins, and such extremes should be avoided. It should be noted that warming an entire bag of blood is fraught with difficulties due to uneven heating and the possibility of overheating; hence in-line (post-bag) warming is the only method widely recommended now.

$$\text{Shear Stress} \propto \text{Yield Stress} + \text{Viscosity Function} \times \text{Shear Rate}$$

or

$$\tau^{1/2} = \tau_y^{1/2} + S^2 Y^{1/2}$$

Figure 4. Casson model for blood rheology.

Rheologic Factors

A number of mechanical factors play significant roles in destruction of cellular components during the transfusion process. These factors, which can be divided into intracellular and extracellular variables, are directly influenced by the amount of energy and momentum contained within the blood as it flows through the transfusion delivery system (see Fig. 2). Extracellular factors are defined by rheology, the study of forces in complex flow states. The external forces which act upon blood constituents result directly from the rheologic properties (which describe the flow characteristics) of the fluid.[4]

A RHEOLOGIC PRIMER

Blood is a very complex fluid, comprising a liquid phase (plasma) and a particulate phase (cellular constituents). Blood flowing in a tube behaves more like India ink than like water. Let us look at the terms and concepts which describe these differences.

Because of differing rheologic properties, water is considered to be close to ideal, or Newtonian, in character, while the more complex fluid, blood, is called non-Newtonian. This means that the behavior of

$$\text{Shear Stress} \propto \text{Yield Stress} + \text{Viscosity Function} \times \text{Velocity Gradient Function}$$

or

$$\tau^{1/2} = f_1 (\text{Hct, Protein Conc.})^{1/2} + f_2 (\mu p \text{ Hct, Protein Conc.}) \times f_3 (\text{flowrate})$$

Figure 5. Determinants of shear stress.

Shear Stress → Hemolysis → Plasma Free
on RBC   Hemoglobin

Figure 6. Effects of shear stress on red blood cells.

blood, because of its complex composition, is described by a complex mathematical model called the Casson model (Fig. 4). Briefly, this model states that the resultant force acting on cellular constituents (shear stress) (Fig. 5), is directly proportional to the degree of aggregation, or amount of force, required to get the flow started (yield stress). Shear stress is also proportional to the resistance of the fluid to flow (viscosity). The damaging force (shear stress) is proportional to the abrupt changes in velocity produced by flowing through a particular apparatus (summarized by "rate of shear"). These velocity gradients may not occur uniformly from side to side in a tube, but may vary with distance from the center.

Workers within the field of materials fabrication for blood flow systems (heart-lung, hemodialysis, blood transfusion) have noted that the amount of cellular destruction is directly proportional to the amount of mechanical shear stress.[5] Hence, any factor that produces an increase in shear stress also increases the amount of cellular damage (e.g., red cell hemolysis) (Fig. 6). It follows that any factor which causes an increase in yield stress, viscosity, or rate of shear likewise increases shear stress (and thus cellular damage).

Yield stress, viscosity, and shear rate are directly affected by the properties of blood components, hematocrit, protein concentration, and flow rate. As shown in Figure 7, yield stress is a direct function of the concentration of the cellular constituents (such as red blood cell (RBC) hematocrit) and of the plasma proteins. Viscosity is a direct function of the viscosity of plasma, the particulate matter concentration (such as RBC hematocrit), and the plasma protein concentration. Shear rate (velocity gradient) is primarily a function of flow rate and the characteristics of the flow, that is, laminar or turbulent.

$$\text{Yield Stress} = \tau_y \, \alpha \, f_1 \, (\text{Hct, Protein Conc.})$$

$$\text{Viscosity Function} = S^2 \, \alpha \, f_2 \, (\mu p, \text{Hct, Protein Conc.})$$

$$\text{Shear Rate} = \gamma \, \alpha \, dv/dy \, \alpha \, \bar{f}_3 \, (\text{flowrate, velocity gradient})$$

Figure 7. Determinants of rheologic properties.

PRACTICAL CONSIDERATIONS

OTHER EQUIPMENT CONSIDERATIONS

We have shown that increases in shear stress significantly increase the creation of cellular debris, and that the apparatus used has a significant effect upon shear stress. Apparatus effects are related primarily to flow rate. Since the flow through most of the blood infusion set is laminar in nature (that is, the flow has a Reynolds number of less than 2100), the rate of flow is a function of the resistance of the transfusion system. Resistance, in turn, varies inversely with the fourth power of the radius and directly with the viscosity and length of tubing. The flow also varies directly with the effects of the driving force (or pressure). For example, the greater the force exerted by a pressure bag or in-line pump, the higher the flow. Increase in the length of tubing utilized in the transfusion apparatus proportionately increases the resistance, hence decreasing flow. Another factor which may sharply decrease flow is decreasing radius of the tubing, owing to the fourth-power relationship.

A typical method by which blood is transfused begins by adding a filter to the transfusion system. Packed red blood cells are attached to the filter, and usually 200 ml normal saline is added through a Y-connection to the bag, and the bag gently agitated. The bag containing the diluted packed cells is placed in a pressure bag (pump), and a pressure of 250 to 300 mmHg applied. From the microaggregate filter, the blood passes to the infusion set, which contains a 170-μm filter. The blood may pass through a heater (one using a length of tubing in a waterbath, or one with a thin-wall bag and an expanded surface area in a dry heater), through various lengths of tubing, and finally may be piggybacked into an IV or into the patient through a separate catheter. The flow rate is directly affected by increasing resistance. Flow rates can drop from a high of 200 ml per minute to 35 to 40 ml per minute, depending upon the apparatus utilized.[6]

However, it should be noted that blood filters are designed and utilized improperly in most cases: smaller size microfilters (20 and 40 μm) are placed upstream of the 170-μm filter, that is, between the unit of blood and the coarser filter. Hence, the life and efficiency of filters is decreased due to clogging by large particles which could have been trapped by the coarse filter.

In addition to decreasing the flow rate, each component utilized also has a potential for increasing mechanical shear stress applied by the apparatus. This is discussed below.

Filters

Various combinations of filters have been employed to remove debris associated with stored blood. However, the rationale for utilization of filters during transfusion of blood products is beyond the scope of this chapter. The existence of microaggregates in blood is well established, but the need for their removal remains controversial. Because administering a transfusion usually requires some sort of filter, the effects of filters upon the cellular constituents should be considered.

Most blood filters are of three basic types: the 170-μm macrofilter, constructed of plastic screen; the 40-μm screen filter, made of metal or plastic screen with high surface area; and 20-μm depth filters, made of Dacron or wool packed in a chamber.

The clinical value of a filter results from the efficiency with which it removes aggregates of various sizes, but when large volumes of blood replacement are required, no filter should be used if it significantly reduces the rate of flow.[7] Buley and Lumley[8] compared the rate of filtration when successive units of blood were run through various types of filters under pressure. They found that the filtration efficiency and rate varied among filter types. There was no consistency as to how many units one filter would tolerate before losing efficiency or flow rate among different makes of filters.

Morphologic changes in red cells and other cellular components are known to result from blood storage. When red cells pass through a filter under pressure, increasing damage may occur, as measured by changes in levels of plasma hemoglobin after filtration. The study by Buley and Lumley demonstrated that when blood that had been stored for periods of less than one week was used, increases in free hemoglobin were small with all types of filters. However, using units that had been stored for up to three weeks, only depth filters (those using Dacron, wool, or other filaments) produced large amounts of free hemoglobin. Hemolysis was not noted after filtration through other types of filters. Cullen and Ferrara[9] have shown that infusing nonexpired whole blood, or fresh-frozen or refrigerated erythrocytes through fine screen filters at 300 mmHg, is efficacious and safe. Cell counts, hematocrit, and free hemoglobin were essentially unchanged.

Gervin and associates[10] demonstrated that coagulation and fibrinolytic mechanisms in both stored blood and fresh frozen blood remain unaltered by microfiltration. They also showed that platelet function was not affected. However, investigation revealed that the number of platelets was reduced in both types of blood by passage through a depth filter. Other workers, such as Snyder's group,[11] have reported that a significant reduction in 22°C stored platelets was not found using 170-μm, 40-μm, or 20-μm filters.

There appears to be no significant clinical experience or other evidence that infusion of particles smaller than 40 μm is harmful to health.[7] Forty-μm screen filters remove large amounts of aggregates, and have been shown to remove the largest volume of debris. This type of filter allows unimpeded passage of a large number of units of blood (greater than 10) without damage to red blood cells.

HOW DO WE GIVE COMPONENTS?

Red Blood Cells

Component therapy, rather than whole blood, has become the mainstay of blood transfusion. We must ensure that red blood cells survive the transfusion process so the patient can use them. The physical integrity of packed red blood cells, like all constituents, is affected by physical forces acting upon them (rheologic forces). Anesthesiologists are recurrently faced with a dilemma: How should packed RBC be transfused to reduce erythrocyte damage (hemolysis) while increasing the flow rate? Since shear stress on the red blood cells produces hemolysis, we must somehow reduce this stress.

The shear stress (and hence the amount of hemolysis, see Fig. 6) is related to the hematocrit, protein concentration, and flow rate. These variables are functions of dilution and rate of administration through a particular apparatus. RBC hemolysis also occurs from mechanical shear stress produced by synthetic materials incompatible with the cells. However, a gap exists between available information regarding RBC shear stress and application to clinical transfusion. Prospective, randomized measurement was made of the independent and interactional effects of dilution, pressure, and apparatus on red cell hemolysis and flow rate.[6] This study showed that regardless of the external pressure applied or the transfusion apparatus used, packed red blood cells should be diluted to decrease hemolysis and increase flow rate. If undiluted packed red blood cells are transfused, there is a risk of increased mechanical damage by known rheologic factors (shear stress). Such damage will result in an increase in free hemoglobin concentration, which may be detrimental to organ systems such as the hepatic and renal systems. Although packed red blood cell flow rate is determined by dilution, pressure, and apparatus, no correlation was found between flow rate and hemolysis.

What agent should be used to dilute the packed red blood cells? As was shown in Figure 2, mechanical factors include intracellular factors which are determined by osmotic gradients. Work by Jones, Kilpatrick, and Franks[2] has demonstrated that to maintain cell viability, isotonic solutions, particularly normal saline, should be utilized. Nonisotonic solutions present problems. Hypotonicity causes water imbalance and increases in cell volume with resultant cellular destruction. Hypertonic solutions produce the opposite effect. Because of the osmotic imbalance, the cells shrink in volume and are agglutinated, as discussed above. Some hypertonic solutions are solutions with 5 percent dextrose, such as D5 Ringer's lactate, and so forth.

Ringer's lactate and other calcium-containing solutions also add another undesirable factor to red blood cells. Calcium will antagonize the various citrate anticoagulant solutions by overcoming the chelating power of citrate. Hence, the citrate will be ineffective and blood may coagulate.

Platelets

Platelets are much smaller cellular constituents than packed red blood cells. Rheologically, platelets behave in a manner similar to red blood cells. Temperature and filtration, as well as types of materials utilized, play important roles in the viability as well as the number of platelets the patient receives. Should platelets be filtered? Recent work by Snyder and associates[11] has indicated that as long as platelets stored at 22°C and previously unused microaggregate filters are used, the activity and number of platelets are not decreased. However, care should be taken when using platelets stored at 4°C since adhesive properties (or stickiness) of platelets stored at this temperature are greatly increased.[12]

Fresh Frozen Plasma and Clotting Concentrates

Filtration of fresh frozen plasma and clotting concentrates has been recommended in the past primarily because of particulate matter they may contain. This advice remains valid.

SUMMARY

A wide selection of blood administration equipment is available from many manufacturers. It would be inappropriate to comment on relative merits of specific brands or types of equipment, since changes in product lines are announced monthly, and one lot of supplies received by a hospital may differ from another. It is important to consider the recommendations made in this chapter when purchasing equipment. When confronted by a manufacturer's representative, the anesthesiologist is well advised to ask for information concerning mechanical factors that may adversely affect the blood's rheologic properties. With respect to filters, it is prudent to inquire not only about their filtration efficiency, but also about their capacity for particulate matter, their effect on red blood cells and platelets, and their ability to sustain high flow rates when massive transfusion is necessary.

In-line blood pumps must be evaluated for evidence of increased shear stress and ease of use. Stopcocks, intravenous catheters, and other areas of constriction along the path of the blood may cause increases in shear stress because of poor design, and resistance may also increase due to small constrictions.

Blood warmers deserve special attention because of the several competing types on the market. In addition to cost and ease of use, reliability, fail-safe mechanisms to avoid overheating of blood, minimum resistance to flow, and large capacity for heat transfer in case of massive transfusion must all be ascertained before purchase. If possible, data should be obtained from independent sources documenting performance of a blood warmer before purchase is considered.

Use of these guidelines, will permit consideration of factors other than price and convenience when selecting materials and methods for safe, convenient transfusion of blood and its components. As more data become available concerning relationships between transfusion equipment, techniques, and preservation of blood components, the anesthesiologist will be better able to make choices based on sound knowledge and experience.

REFERENCES

1. VALERI, RC AND HIRSCH, NM: *Restoration in vivo of erythrocyte adenosine triphosphate, 2,3-diphosphoglycerate, potassium ion and sodium concentrations following the transfusion of acid-citrate-dextrose-stored human red blood cells.* J Lab Clin Med 73:722, 1969.

2. JONES, JH, KILPATRICK, GS, and FRANKS, EH: *Red cell aggregation in dextrose solutions.* J Clin Path 15:161, 1962.
3. BOYAN, CP: *Cold or warmed blood for massive transfusions?* Ann Surg 160:282, 1964.
4. GORDON, RJ and RAVIN, MB: *Rheology and anesthesiology.* Anesth Analg 57:252, 1978.
5. KELLER, KH, ET AL: *Guidelines for Blood-Material Interactions.* NIH Publication #80-2185. National Institutes of Health, Bethesda, Maryland, 1980.
6. CALKINS, JM, ET AL: *Critical importance of diluting packed RBC for transfusion.* Anesthiology (Suppl) 53:S169, 1980.
7. WALKER, AKY: *Blood microfiltration.* Anaesthesia 33:35, 1978.
8. BULEY, R AND LUMLEY, J: *Some observations on blood microfilters.* Ann Royal Col Surg Eng 57:262, 1975.
9. CULLEN, DJ and FERRARA, LC: *Fine-screen filtration of pressurized whole blood, packed cells, and fresh-frozen erythrocytes.* Anesthesiology 43:578, 1975.
10. GERVIN, AS, ET AL: *Ultrapore hemofiltration: The effects on the coagulation and fibrinolytic mechanisms in fresh and stored blood.* Arch Surg 106:333, 1973.
11. SNYDER, EL, ET AL: *Transfusion of platelets through microaggregate filters.* Anesthesiology (Suppl) 51:S205, 1979.
12. HUESTIS, DW, BOVE, JR, AND BUSCH, S: *Practical Blood Transfusion,* ed 2. Little, Brown & Co, Boston, 1976, p 78.

INDEX

ACID-BASE imbalance
  in massive transfusion, 161
Acute respiratory distress syndrome
  comparison of the effects of balanced salt solution vs. albumin on, 65-68
Albumin
  advantages of, 124
  effect of infusions, 127
Albumin solutions
  comparison of, with balanced salt solutions, 60-69
    clinical studies
      cost, 69
      extracellular fluid changes, 61-65
      hepatic function, 69
      pulmonary consequences of shock and resuscitation, 65-68
      renal responses, 68-69
Alloxan, 110-111
American Association of Blood Banks, 158
Anemia, correction of, 152, 157
Antidiuretic hormone (ADH), 43-45, 89-90
Azotemia, 145, 147

BALANCED salt solutions in massive trauma
  choices of solutions, 72-73
  comparison of, with albumin solutions, 60-69
    clinical studies, 69-72
    cost, 69
    extracellular fluid changes, 61-65
    hepatic function, 69
    pulmonary consequences, 65-68
    renal response, 68-69
  intravascular fluid loss and
    mechanisms of, 59
    physiologic response to, 59-60
  shock and, 58-59
  therapy for
    evaluation of, 76-79
    postresuscitation hypertension and, 79-80
    principles of, 74-75
    regimen for, 75-76
Balanced salt solutions as renal prophylaxis *See also* Renal insufficiency.
  administration of, 140-141
  and hypothermia, 140

183

Balanced salt solutions—*Continued*
  in surgery, 140
  and tissue damage, 141–142
  and urine output, 140
  following surgery and trauma
    clinical studies, 143–146
  function of, 139
  in nonoliguric renal failure
    clinical course of, 147
    frequency of, 147
    mortality in, 147
  in oliguric renal failure
    clinical course of, 149
    dialysis in, choice of procedure, 149
    hazards in surgery, 149
Baroreceptors
  influence on ADH release, 44–45
Bernard, Claude, 6
Bleeding in surgery, 162–164
Blood
  banked, 160–161
  crossmatching, 156
  in hemorrhagic shock, 76
Blood components, 154–155, *t*
  proper methods for warming, 173
  risks of damage to, 178–179
Blood component therapy. *See also* Blood components.
  advantages of, 151
  bleeding problems and, 153, 156
  components, use of, *t*, 154–155
  crossmatching, use of, 156
  preoperative transfusion
    to correct anemia, 152
    patient reaction to, 153
    timing of, 153
  red cells, use of
    advantages over whole blood, 157
    disadvantages of, 157
  surgical bleeding
    causes of, 162–163
    treatment of, 163–164
  transfusion in surgery
    excessive blood loss, 158
    hemodilution, effect of, 158
    massive, 160–162
      defective hemostasis in, 160
      problems associated with, 161–162
  whole blood
    problems associated with, 156–157
Blood filters, 176–177
  effects of filtration, 177–178
Blood pressure
  effect of decreased intravascular volume on, 59
Blood substitutes, risks of, 73–74
Blood products
  and component viability, 170, *f*
  and osmotic factors, 171–173
  and physical factors, 171–175
  and rheologic factors, 174–175
  and temperature factors, 173
Blood substitutes
  comparison of, 73–74
Blood transfusion
  during surgery, 158–160
  massive, 160–162
  preoperative, 152–156
    precautions in, 156
    reactions to, 153
Blood warmers, 160
BSS. *See* Balanced salt solutions.

CAPACITANCE shock, 58
Capillary filtration coefficient. *See* Colloid osmotic pressure in shock resuscitation.
Cardiac surgery
  and alterations in hemostasis, 164
Cardiogenic shock, 58
Casson model, 174, *f*, 175
Central venous pressure (CVP)
  measurement of, 77–78
Citrate toxicity, 161
Coagulation factor deficiencies
  in surgery, 164
Colloid osmotic pressure in shock
  and capillary filtration coefficient
    clinical studies of, 104
    and lymph flow rate, 104–105
    measurement of, 103–104
    edema safety factor in, 109–112
    measurement of, 109
    and plasma oncotic pressure, *f*, 110, 112
    effect on edema, 111
    vs. cricital capillary pressure, *f*, 111
  and lymph flow
    clinical studies, 108–109
  and lung permeability
    clinical studies, 113–115
    effect of increase in, 110–112

and pulmonary capillary pressure
   clinical studies, 107
   measurement of, 107
and tissue fluid pressure
   hydrostatic pressure, 106
   oncotic pressure, 105–106
and transcapillary fluid exchange
   clinical tests for permeability, 103
   measurement of, 102
Colloid oncotic pressure
   clinical studies, 128–130
     studies in baboons, 128
     studies in sheep, 127
   effect of, f, 126
   effects of changes in, 125–127, 128–131
Consumptive coagulopathy, 163

Danang lung, 101
Deoxycorticosterone acetate (DOCA), f, 41
Dextran
   disadvantages of, 74, 158
Dextrose
   use in solutions, 14–15
Dialysis. *See* Renal failure, oliguric.
Drugs
   with antidiuretic properties, t, 48

Edema
   and hyponatremia, 46
   and surgical operations, 1–31
   and trauma, 1–31
   Edema, history of, 1–31
     distant history (1900–1939), 7–10
     modern history (1950–Present), 11–14
     recent history (1940–1950,) 10–11
     remote history (1628–1899), 3–7
Edema safety factor. *See* Colloid osmotic pressure in shock.
Electrolyte solutions, 72–73
Endotoxin, 112
Equipment. *See also* filters.
   in transfusion
Extracellular fluid volume
   comparison of effects of balanced salt solutions vs. albumin on, 61–65

Fasting. *See also* Preoperative preparation.
   complications of, 91

Filters. *See also* Transfusion during anesthesia.
   in blood transfusion, 159
Fluid administration
   following surgery, 129
   recommended regimen, 14–15
     in extremities and major superficial operations, 15
     in intra-abdominal and hip operations, 14
     in intracranial procedures, 15
     in intrathoracic operations, 15
     in microsurgery of the ear and larnyx, 15
     in most opthalmic operations, 15
     in transurethral prostatic surgery, 15
Fluid loss
   in massive trauma, 58–59
   compensatory mechanisms for, 89
   physiologic response to, 59–60
   preoperative, 89–90
   secondary to massive trauma, 59
   signs of, 89
Fluid therapy, intraoperative in pediatrics
   evaluation of patient, 87–90
     effects of fasting (NPO), 88
     fluid states prior to surgery
       definitive compensatory mechanisms for, 90
       temporary compensatory mechanisms for, 89
     need for IV, 91
       adverse effects of fluids, 92
       choice of fluids, 91–92, 98
     results of diagnostic studies, 88
   goals of therapy, 92–94
     guidelines for fluid administration, 92–93
     to ensure hydration, 93
     to replace blood loss, 94
   intraoperative hypotension
     causes of, 95–96
     therapy for, 96
   patient monitoring, techniques of, 95
Fluid therapy in post-traumatic respiratory failure
   choice of fluids, 123–124, 127–128
   dynamics of fluid exchanges
     effects of albumin, 127–128
     changes in permeability, 127
     clinical studies, 125, 127, 128–129
     in injury and sepsis, 126–127

Fluid therapy in post-traumatic respiratory failure—*Continued*
  guidelines for therapy
    choice of fluid regimen, 131
    measurement of results, 131–132
  respiratory distress syndrome (ARDS)
    causes of, 121
    clinical studies, 121–122
    fluid overload in, 121
    sepsis in, 122–123
Fluid volume
  extracellular
    comparison of effects of balanced salt
    solutions vs. albumin on, 61–65
Furosemide
  in treatment of hyponatremia, *f*, 51

Harvey, William, 2,3
Heart rate
  effect of decreased intravascular volume on, 59
Hemodilution
  during surgery, 158
Hemodynamic monitoring. *See* Monitoring.
Hemorrhagic shock, 61–65, 68–69
  animal studies of, 62–65
  renal responses in, 68–69
Henle's loop, 36, 39–40, 44
Historical aspects of
  anesthesia, 10–12
    effects on renal function and salt solutions, 10–11
      caution against, 10
      and postmortem findings, 11
      successful use of, 12
  extracellular fluid (ECF), 2
    loss of in shock, 13–14
  hypodermic medication, 6
  intravenous injection, 3–9
    of acacia
      and bacterial contamination, 8–9
    of drugs, 3–4
    methods and techniques of, 9
    of salt solutions, 7–8
      criticism of, 8
      and infant diarrhea, 5
Hepatic function
  comparison of the effects of balanced salt solutions vs. albumin on, 69
Hyperglycemia, 92

Hypernatremia
  causes of, 52–53
  mortality in, 52–53
  symptoms of, 52
  treatment of, 53–54
Hypertension
  postresuscitation, 79–80
Hypoalbuminemia, 64
Hypoglycemia, 92
Hyponatremia
  acute, 49
  and antidiuretic drugs, *t*, 48
  causes of, *t*, 47
Hyponatremia
  diagnosis of, 45–48
  differential diagnosis, 48
  and edema, 46
  mortality in, 49
  and serum osmolality, 45
    calculation of, 45–46
  signs and symptoms of, 48
  treatment of, 49–52
    by fluid restriction, 50
    with sodium, 49
Hypoperfusion
  definition of, 58
Hypotension, intraoperative, 95–96
  causes of, 96
  correction of, 96
Hypothermia
  use in surgery, 140–141
Hypovolemic shock, 59–80. *See also,* Shock.
  central venous pressure in, 77
  extracellular fluid changes in, 61–65
  intravascular fluid loss in, 59–60
  pulmonary consequences of, 65–68
    acute respiratory distress in, 65, 67
    lymphatic system, function of, 66, 68
  resuscitative fluid used in, 60–74
  treatment of, 74–80

Intraoperative fluid therapy, 91–94
  and hyperalimentation fluids, 92
  and hyperglycemia, 92
  and hypoglycemia, 92
  and nontraumatic surgery, 92
  and patient monitoring, 95
  and surgical trauma, 91
Intravascular volume
  decrease in
    physiologic response to, 59–60

Intravenous fluid administration
 history of, 1–31
 saline solutions, 5, 7, 10
Intravenous injection
 history of, 3–31
Isotopes, use of
 in measuring extracellular volume, 60–61

KIDNEY
 evolution of, 34–35
 normal function of, 35–36
 physiology of, f, 34
 vasculotubular relationships of, f, 36

LIVER disease
 problem in surgery, 163
Lung
 effect of resuscitation on, 67–68
 fluid exchanges in shock, 102–103
 measurement of, 102
 permeability changes in, 110–115
 permeability studies of, 103–104, 106–107, 113–115
 pressure changes in, 102–110
Lymphatic system
 function of, 66

MANNITOL, 140
Mineralcorticoids, importance of, 41
Monitoring
 of patient response to therapy in hypovolemic shock, 77–79
 techniques of, 95
Moyer, Carl A, 5, 10–12
Myoglobinuria, 140

NATRIURETIC hormone, 42
Nephron
 classes of, 35
 transport processes of, f, 38
Normal saline. See also Balanced salt solutions.
 comparison of, with Ringer's lactate, 72–73

PEEP. See positive end expiratory pressure.
Plasma, human
 risks of, 73
Platelet count
 significance in surgical bleeding, 163

Platelet function
 defects in surgery, 164
Platelets, storage and filtering of, 179
Positive end expiratory pressure (PEEP)
 therapeutic use of, 131–132
Postoperative period
 fluid management in children, 97–98
 tissue trauma in, 97
 urine output in, 97
Postresuscitation hypertension, 79–80
Preoperative preparation
 and fasting, 88
 fluid loss in, 89–90
 of pediatric patients, 87–91
 problems in children, 88
Protein factions
 and tissue fluid oncotic pressure, 105–106, 109
Potassium toxicity
 in massive transfusion, 161
Pseudohyponatremia, 45
Pulmonary artery exclusion pressure
 measurement of, 131–132
Pulmonary capillary pressure, 107–108
Pulmonary edema, 102–115
Pulmonary insufficiency. See also Respiratory distress syndrome.
 fluid regimen for, 123–128
 mortality rates for, 120
 pathogenesis of, 120–122
Pulmonary lymph flow, 108–109
Pulmonary safety factor, 109, 125

RAA. See Renin-angiotensin-aldosterone system
Red blood cells
 advantages of, 157
 damaged by storage, 171
 protection from damage, 172–173
 restoration of, 171
Reflection coefficient, 108
Renal circulation, 36–37
Renal damage
 following injury and shock, 143–146
 sodium balance in, 145–146
 urea clearance in, 143
Renal failure, nonoliguric, 147–148
 clinical course of, 147
 factors in, 148
 frequency of, 147
 mortality rate for, 147

Renal failure, oliguric, 148–150
  peritoneal dialysis in, 150
  prophylactic dialysis in, 149
  surgical procedures in, 149
Renal function
  after trauma, 144–145
  comparison of the effects of balanced salt solutions vs. albumin on, 65–68
  in the infant, 86–87
  studies of, 143
  variables of, 87
Renal insufficiency
  incidence of, 138
  prevention of, 138–139
  treatment of, 140–142
Renal responses
  following surgery and trauma, 143–150
Renin-angiotensin-aldosterone (RAA) system
  function of, 90
  and release of ADH, 90
  signs of activation of, 90
Respiratory distress syndrome (ARDS). *See also* Pulmonary insufficiency.
  causes of, 121
  effect of, 121
  factors in, 123
  fluid overload in, 121
  sepsis in, 122
Resuscitative fluid, choice of, 60–72
  albumin solutions, 67–72, 74, 80
  colloid solutions, 66
  crystalloid solutions, 67
  dextran, 74
  Ringer's solution, 72–73, 75–76
Rheologic factors
  in transfusion, 174–175
Ringer's lactate
  comparison with albumin, 124
  early use of, 12
  in hemorrhagic shock, 64
  in hypovolemic shock, 60, 72–73, 75–76
  as substitute for blood, 119

SALT
  tolerance in infants, 85
Salt solutions. *See* Balanced salt solutions.
Serum osmolality, 45–46
Shear stress in blood flow, 175–176
  effect on red blood cells, 175, *f,* 178

Shock. *Also see* Colloid osmotic pressure in shock.
  capacitance, 58
  cardiogenic, 58
  definition of, 58
  fluid loss during, 62, 75
  hypovolemic, 58–80
Sodium
  retention in hyponatremia, 46
  in treatment of hyponatremia, 49–50
Sodium balance. *See also* Sodium excretion and sodium reabsorption.
  and Henle's loop, 39–40
  and hydrostatic pressure, 37
  and medullary blood flow, 42
  and renal circulation, 36–37
  and Starling's forces
    role in sodium reabsorption, 42
  and tubular function, 37–40
Sodium excretion, 40–42. *See also* Sodium reabsorption.
  mechanisms controlling, 40–43
  deoxycorticosterone acetate (DOCA), 41
  DOCA escape phenomenon, *f,* 41
  glomerular filtration rate, 40, 42
  mineralcorticoids
  natriuretic hormone, 42
  sympathetic nerve activity, 43
Sodium reabsorption, 40–43. *See also* Sodium excretion.
  and distribution of blood flow, 42–43
  and medullary blood flow, 42
  and Starling's forces, 42
Starling equation, 102, 109, 124
Starling's forces, 38, 42, 44
Starling's Law, 66
Stored blood, problems of, 162
Swan-Ganz catheter, 78–79, 95, 125
Syndrome(s)
  acute respiratory distress
  comparison of the effects of balanced salt solutions vs. albumin on, 65–68

THERAPY
  in hypovolemic shock
    evaluation of, 76–79
    postresuscitation hypertension and, 79–80
    principles of, 74–75
    regimen for, 75–76

Thrombocytopenia
  in surgery, 164
Tissue fluid hydrostatic pressure, 106
Tissue fluid oncotic pressure, 105–106
Transfusion
  and hemodilution, 158
  in surgery, 158–162
  massive, 160–162
  preoperative, 152–153
Transfusion delivery system, 171, f
Transfusion during anesthesia
  damage to red blood cells- 178–179
  platelets, use of, 179
  physical factors affecting, 171–178
    osmotic factors
      prevention of damage by, 172–173
      problems associated with, 171–172
    rheologic factors
      description of,174–175
    temperature factors
      extremes to be avoided, 173
    transfusion systems
      filters used in, 176–177
Trauma
  and isolated lung preparations, 104
  to tissue, 97
    fluids used in, 97

Trauma, massive. *See also,* Shock, hypovolemic.
  blood loss in, 76–77
  clinical studies of, 69–72
  and fluid balance, 57–80
  and intravascular fluid loss, 59–60
  initial treatment of, 75
  lymph flow in, 66
  measurement of fluid losses in, 61–62
  and pulmonary edema, 67–68
  response to treatment, 78
Treatment. *See* Therapy.
Tubular function
  mechanisms of, 37–40
  normal, 35–40

Urine
  concentration and dilution of, 43–45
    and ADH release, 44
      mechanisms for, 44–45
    and acute renal failure, 44
    factors necessary for, 43
    and hyponatremia, 45
    and hypotension, 44
    and water deprivation, 43

Vasopressin, effects of, 90

Whole blood, use of, 156–157